DUAL DIAGNOSIS

SUBSTANCE MISUSE AND PSYCHIATRIC DISORDERS

Edited by

G. HUSSEIN RASSOOL

MSc, BA, RN, FETC, RCNT, RNT , MILT, FRSH
Cert. Ed., Cert. Couns., Cert. in Supervision & Consultation.
Senior Lecturer/Course Leader — Dual Diagnosis Module and Msc in Addictive Behaviour
Department of Addictive Behaviour & Psychological Medicine
Centre for Addiction Studies
St George's Hospital Medical School (University of London),UK

Visiting Professor São Paulo University, Brazil

**Blackwell
Science**

DISTRIBUTORS
Marston Book Services Ltd
PO Box 269
Abingdon
Oxon OX14 4YN
(Orders: Tel: 01235 465500
         Fax: 01235 465555)

USA
Blackwell Science, Inc.
Commerce Place
350 Main Street
Malden, MA 02148 5018
(Orders: Tel: 800 759 6102
               781 388 8250
         Fax: 781 388 8255)

Canada
Login Brothers Book Company
324 Saulteaux Crescent
Winnipeg, Manitoba R3J 3T2
(Orders: Tel: 204 837 3987
         Fax: 204 837 3116)

Australia
Blackwell Science Pty Ltd
54 University Street
Carlton, Victoria 3053
(Orders: Tel: 03 9347 0300
         Fax: 03 9347 5001)

A catalogue record for this title
is available from the British Library

ISBN 0-632-05621-5

Library of Congress
Cataloging-in-Publication Data

Dual diagnosis, substance misuse and psychiatric
disorders / edited by G. Haussein Rassool.
        p.   ;   cm.
    Includes bibliographical references and index.
    ISBN 0-632-05621-5 (alk. paper)
    1. Dual diagnosis. I. Rassool, G. Hussein.
    [DNLM: 1. Substance-Related Disorders—
diagnosis.   2. Diagnosis, Dual (Psychiatry).
3. Mental Disorders—complications. 4. Mental
Disorders—diagnosis. 5. Mental Disorders—
therapy. 6. Substance-Related Disorders—
complications. 7. Substance-Related
Disorders—therapy. WM 270 D8128 2001]
RC564.68. D795 2001
616.86′075—dc21

                                    2001035734

Dedicated to Julie, Yasmin Soraya, Adam Ali Hussein, Reshad Hassan, and Hassim Rassool

Contents

Contributors

Mohammad Abou-Saleh   *Clinical Director South West London and St George's Mental Health NHS Trust, Substance Misuse Services/Reader. Department of Addictive Behaviour & Psychological Medicine. Centre for Addiction Studies, St George's Hospital Medical School (University of London). London.*

Ken Checinski   *Consultant Psychiatrist Surrey Oaklands NHS Trust, Community Drug and Alcohol Team/Senior Lecturer. Department of Addictive Behaviour Psychological Medicine. Centre for Addiction Studies, St George's Hospital Medical School (University of London). London.*

James Edeh   *Consultant Psychiatrist, Mid Sussex NHS Trust, Substance Misuse Services/Senior Lecturer. Department of Addictive Behaviour & Psychological Medicine. Centre for Addiction Studies, St George's Hospital Medical School (University of London). London.*

Mike Flanagan   *Clinical Advice/Service Development Co-ordinator. Addictions Resource Agency for Commissioners (ARAC) Department of Addictive Behaviour & Psychological Medicine, St George's Hospital Medical School (University of London). London.*

Charlotte Harrison   *Specialist Senior Registrar in Addiction. Department of Addictive Behaviour & Psychological Medicine. Centre for Addiction Studies, St George's Hospital Medical School (University of London). London.*

Alison Keating   *Policy Analyst/Senior Social Worker. Addictions Resource Agency for Commissioners (ARAC) Department of Addictive Behaviour & Psychological Medicine, St George's Hospital Medical School (University of London). London.*

Alison Lowe   *Consultant Psychiatrist. Haringey Healthcare NHS Trust, Dual Diagnosis Service. Dual Diagnosis Service, St Ann's Hospital. London.*

Kim Moore   *Senior Addiction Nurse. Dual Diagnosis Service, St Ann's Hospital. London.*

Adenekan Oyefeso   *Senior Lecturer/Consultant Psychologist. Department of Addictive Behaviour & Psychological Medicine. Centre for Addiction Studies, St George's Hospital Medical School (University of London). London.*

Contributors

Peter Price   *Senior Lecturer. Faculty of Health and Social Care Sciences, Kingston University & St George's Hospital Medical School (University of London). London.*

Salman Rawaf   *Consultant Public Health Physician. Director of Clinical Standards, Merton, Sutton & Wandsworth Health Authority, Mitcham, London.*

G. Hussein Rassool   *Senior Lecturer & Course Leader Msc in Addictive Behaviour. Department of Addictive Behaviour & Psychological Medicine. Centre for Addiction Studies, St George's Hospital Medical School (University of London). London.*

Fred Roach   *Consultant Forensic Clinical Psychologist. Surrey Oaklands NHS Trust. Psychology Department, West Park Hospital, Surrey.*

Daisy Saffer   *Consultant Psychiatrist/Psychotherapist. Surrey Oaklands NHS Trust, Greenbank Substance Misuse Recovery Unit, West Park Hospital, Epsom, Surrey.*

Vivienne Saunders   *Senior Addiction Prevention Practitioner. Department of Addictive Behaviour & Psychological Medicine. Centre for Addiction Studies, St George's Hospital Medical School (University of London). London.*

Fabrizio Schifano   *Former Consultant Psychiatrist, Partita IVA Ospedale dei Colli, Servizio Per Le Tossicodipendence, Padova, Italy. Now, Consultant Psychiatrist Richmond Healthcare Hamlet and Senior Lecturer, Department of Addictive Behaviour & Psychological Medicine, Centre for Addiction Studies, St George's Hospital Medical School (University of London). London.*

Hugh Williams   *Consultant Psychiatrist. South Downs Health NHS Trust. Substance Misuse Services/Senior Lecturer. Substance Misuse Service, Brighton.*

Preface

The book is about the phenomenon of "dual diagnosis", that is, the concurrent existence in an individual of substance misuse and psychiatric disorder(s) in specialist and non-specialist settings and the way that health care professionals have responded to this new challenge. The theme of the book, which is interwoven in all the chapters, is the multi-professional nature of the work with dual diagnosis patients.

The increase in the number of individuals with substance misuse and psychiatric disorders has attracted considerable interest in recent years but the impact on clinical practice and service development has not yet been observed and there is a paucity of literature, especially in the United Kingdom, on the clinical and practical issues for practitioners both in the mental health and addiction field. However, there seems to be a cultural paradigm shift in terminology from 'Dual Diagnosis' to 'Complex Needs'. This book is designed to bridge this gap. The book, which is practice-based, is written by experienced academics and clinicians from the disciplines of nursing, psychiatry, psychology and social work.

The book aims to provide practitioners with a comprehensive text on the contemporary issues of working with dual diagnosis patients from both clinical and theoretical perspectives. It also aims to foster awareness, knowledge and skills of health care professionals required to respond effectively to patients whom they encounter in their daily practice. The book is a synthesis of the body of knowledge, research and clinical practice within the UK framework of dealing with dual diagnosis.

While the book will address issues related to practitioners in dealing with the comorbidity of substance misuse and psychiatric disorders, it will be of interest and act as an excellent resource for other health and social care professionals who are unfamiliar with the "dual diagnosis" phenomenon. It will be of relevance to students in medicine, nursing, psychology, social work and criminal justice system and those attending postgraduate courses in addiction and mental health studies.

Dual diagnosis, like substance misuse, is not the sole property of one particular discipline. It is everybody's business.

Structure of the Book

Dual Diagnosis—Substance Misuse and Psychiatric Disorders is presented in two sections. Part 1 presents the background in providing an overview of dual diagnosis, the conceptual examination of dual diagnosis and substance misuse and their psychopathology. Concepts, models and theories of substance use and dual diagnosis are presented to provide some contextual background for those who have limited knowledge and understanding of substance use and misuse. A European perspective and a psychological research model in the understanding of complex behaviour are also included. Part 2 deals with the specialist response to dual diagnosis, with reference to shared care approach, nursing, social work and medical response, therapeutic interventions, public health perspective, service provision and professional education.

Acknowledgements

The learned man who only talks will never penetrate to the inner heart of man.

Saadi of Shiraz

I would like to thank all the contributors, staff at Blackwell Science — Antonia Seymour and Rupal Malde — for their advice, support, and expertise in the preparation of this book. I am also particularly grateful to Professor James P. Smith, Professor J. Akinsanya and Professor A. Hamid Ghodse, and the Florence Nightingale Research Foundation for their guidance in my professional development. My special thanks to all the students on the MSc (Addictive Behaviour) course.

I would also like to acknowledge the contributions of my teachers who enabled me, through my own reflective practices, to follow the Path. To my dear friend Nek, for all his support and encouragement over the years.

Finally, I owe my gratitude to my family. Julie, for her constant support, directly and indirectly, and to my children, Yasmin, Adam and Reshad.

Part 1: Background

1: Dual Diagnosis—an Overview: Fact or Fiction?

Hugh Williams

Introduction

The concept of dual diagnosis is not new. As early as 1993 the American Psychiatric Association (APA 1994) identified dual diagnosis as '. . . one of the major problems confronting the mental health field in the United States'. More recently the subject has been attracting increased attention on this side of the Atlantic.

Concepts and classification

The terms 'dual diagnosis', and 'comorbidity' are now used commonly and interchangeably. In North America the term 'mentally ill chemical abusers' (MIRAs) appears to be favoured. In its broadest context the concept of 'dual diagnosis' or 'comorbidity' refers to coexistence of any psychiatric disorders and substance use disorders in the same individual. In practice the term is often more specifically restricted to include severe mental illness (psychosis, schizophrenia, bipolar affective illness) and substance misuse disorder. El-Guebaly (1990) suggests the term should include two overlapping but discernible groups of patients. One subgroup has, by DSM-III criteria, both a major substance disorder and a major psychiatric illness. The other subgroup use substances in ways that affect the course and treatment of mental illness. Lehman *et al.* (1989) describe the following clinical classifications:

• Primary mental illness with substance misuse. Here the symptoms, sequelae or treatment of the mental illness lead to drug use.

• Substance misuse with psychiatric sequelae. Included here are the acute psychiatric syndromes associated with drug intoxication or withdrawal (e.g. psychosis induced by psycho-stimulants or depression on withdrawal from cocaine).

• Dual primary diagnosis, where the patient suffers from two initially unrelated disorders that may interact to exacerbate each other.

• Common aetiology group, where common underlying factors may predispose to both conditions (e.g. homelessness as a risk factor for both depression and substance misuse).

3

On the other hand, Rostad and Checinski (1996) claim that the term dual diagnosis is misleading and unhelpful. Nevertheless the same authors do concede that, for the moment, the 'label' is useful in so far as it draws attention to 'a real problem which is not being addressed'.

Epidemiology

Despite certain methodological difficulties, especially with earlier studies, as highlighted by a number of authors (Bryant *et al.* 1992; Weiss *et al.* 1992; Smith & Hucker 1994; El-Guebaly 1995), there is now strong research evidence that the rate of substance misuse is substantially higher among the mentally ill compared with the general population. Khalsa *et al.* (1991) found a comorbidity rate (DSM-III-R criteria for current substance abuse and mental disorder) of 39% among attendees at a psychiatric assessment unit. A study (Menezes *et al.* 1996) of 171 inner city London patients in contact with psychiatric services found the one year prevalence rate among subjects with psychotic illness for any substance misuse problem was 36.3% (31.6% alcohol, 15.8% drug). Similarly, there is evidence that among populations of patients with primary substance use disorders psychiatric conditions are common. The National Treatment Outcome Research Study (NTORS) found that 10% of substance misuse patients entering treatment had a psychiatric admission (not related to substance dependence) in the previous two years (Gossop *et al.* 1998). Suicidal thoughts are commonly reported (Gossop *et al.* 1998) by drug dependent patients (29%) in treatment and substance misuse is known to increase by 8–15 fold the risk of suicide (Shaffer *et al.* 1996; Oyefeso *et al.* 1999). Some of this increased risk may be explained by the presence of comorbid psychiatric conditions such as depression or personality disorder in substance misusers (Neeleman & Farrell 1997).

As patients with comorbid conditions (i.e. more than one disorder) may be more likely to seek treatment, data from clinical samples may represent an over-estimation(El-Guebaly 1995). This effect is referred to as the Berkson' bias. Population studies therefore may offer a more accurate and representative data. The Epidemiological Catchment Area (ECA) study (Regier *et al.* 1990), a large American population survey, found a lifetime prevalence rate for substance misuse disorder of 16.7% (13.5% alcohol, 6.1% drug) for the general population. Rates for patients with schizophrenia, affective disorders and anxiety disorders were 47%, 32% and 23.7%, respectively. For persons with any drug (excluding alcohol) disorder more than half (53%) had one other mental disorder most commonly anxiety and affective disorders.

In the United Kingdom (UK), the Office of Population Censuses and Surveys household survey estimated the prevalence of alcohol and drug dependence among the general population to be 5% and 2%, respectively (Farrell *et al.* 1998). Again anxiety and depression were the most common comorbid conditions.

Aetiological theories

Reasons why the mentally ill misuse drugs

Patients with psychiatric illness may use drugs (or choose certain drugs) for the same reasons as the rest of the population do (e.g. get high, to relax, because of increased availability or acceptability, etc.). While this contention may be true, it fails however, to explain the observed increased prevalence of substance use compared to the general population. A number of possible explanations can therefore be advanced. The mentally ill may experience downward drift to poor inner city areas (social drift hypothesis) where drug availability is increased. Drug use may decrease social isolation by enhancing involvement in a subculture or as Mueser *et al.* (1992) frame it 'substance misuse . . . may meet the patients' socio-affiliative need for acceptance and interpersonal contact'. With the advent of deinstitutionalisation, more of the mentally ill (and vulnerable?) may be finding themselves exposed to an increased availability of drugs in the community. Conversely an increased availability of illicit drugs in psychiatric institutions may be a contributory factor (Laurence 1995; Williams & Cohen 2000). The self-medication theory of Khantzian (1985), which suggests that substance use decreases distress caused by psychiatric symptoms, may still retain some credence. For example opiates, cannabis or alcohol may reduce the agitation and anxiety associated with mental illness while stimulants may be used as self-medication for negative symptoms or depression. Psycho-stimulants may help counteract extrapyramidal side-effects of antipsychotic medication (Smith & Hucker 1994) especially akathesia. Finally, a common genetic susceptibility predisposing to both conditions, for example via genes regulating dopamine or serotonin function, may even exist (Kosten & Ziedonis 1997). Mueser *et al.* (1998) have recently critically reviewed the evidence pertaining to some of the aetiological theories for the increased prevalence of substance misuse in patients with severe mental illness.

Clinical implications of dual diagnosis

For patients with a dual diagnosis, each of the comorbid disorders can have important implications for the course and prognosis of the other disorder. Substance misuse can precipitate psychotic illness in those biologically predisposed and is associated with an earlier age onset of illness (El-Guebaly 1990; Mueser *et al.* 1992; McGuire *et al.* 1994). It may modify the clinical presentation of mental illness (Sokolshi *et al.* 1994), exacerbate existing psychotic symptoms (Negrete *et al.* 1986) and interfere with treatment compliance (Pristach & Smith 1990; Kosten & Ziedonis 1997). Substance misuse has been associated with an increased rate of relapse in the chronically mentally ill (Poole & Brabbins 1996) even in the presence of continued compliance with antipsychotic medication (Gupta *et al.* 1996). Mentally ill substance misusers (compared to non-substance misusers) have higher

5

readmission rates and increased use of inpatient services (Menezes *et al.* 1996; Wu *et al.* 1999). Similarly in the case of drug dependence, concurrent psychiatric conditions, for example depression, have been associated with greater illicit drug use while in treatment and a poorer prognosis (Rounsaville *et al.* 1982). The combination of major psychiatric illness and substance misuse is associated (though not necessarily via a direct causative link) with an increased risk of aggressive and violent behaviour (Johns 1998; Scott *et al.* 1999).

Intoxication masquerading as mental illness?

In assessing patients with psychiatric symptoms and substance misuse accurate assessment is essential in planning effective treatment. However, this can be difficult because of the psychomimetic effects of substance misuse. Substance misuse both in intoxication or withdrawal can give rise to a wide range of psychiatric syndromes and transient psychotic states (Poole & Brabbins 1996). For example, in a patient with psychotic symptoms and substance misuse, the psychotic symptoms may occur as a direct effect of the substance(s) use, may be related to an independent functional illness or may be related to a combination of both (Rosenthal & Miner 1997). The complexity relationship between substance use and psychiatric symptomology is further highlighted in Table 1.1 (Crome 1999).

Clinicians who attempt to diagnose mental illness without assessing for substance misuse run a grave risk of misdiagnosis and consequently, mistreatment (Mueser *et al.* 1992). This may be particularly crucial with first episode psychosis where rates of substance misuse are high (Cantwell *et al.* 1999). Indeed it has been claimed that schizophrenia may be over diagnosed in patients for whom the correct diagnosis was psychosis resulting from substance misuse (Cohen 1995). Equally well there is a risk of missing a diagnosis of mental disorder by too readily attributing symptoms solely to drug misuse. The timing of diagnosis is important, as many drugs can produce transient short-lived syndromes which will settle within days to weeks. Clin-

Table 1.1 Substance use and psychiatric syndromes.

Substance use (even single dose) may lead to psychiatric syndromes/symptoms
Harmful use may produce psychiatric syndromes
Dependence may produce psychological symptoms
Intoxication from substances may produce psychological symptoms
Withdrawal from substances may produce psychological symptoms
Withdrawal from substances may lead to psychiatric syndromes
Substance use may exacerbate pre-existing psychiatric disorder
Psychological morbidity not amounting to a disorder may precipitate substance use
Primary psychiatric disorder may lead to substance use disorder
Primary psychiatric disorder may precipitate substance disorder, which may, in turn, lead
   to psychiatric syndromes

Based on Crome (1999).

icians must establish abstinence criteria, i.e. a period of time that the patient must be drug free before a psychiatric disorder, other than a substance use disorder can be diagnosed (Weiss *et al.* 1992; Cohen 1995). The point is well demonstrated in a study by Davidson concerning the diagnosis of depression in alcoholics undergoing detoxification (Davidson 1995). Cohen (1995) asserts that the only way to be sure that psychoactive substances cause illness is if the patient recovers when he/she stops using them. If the symptoms return when the substance use is resumed the diagnosis is confirmed. Mueser *et al.* (1992) maintain that if substance misuse has occurred in the past, but there is clear evidence of schizophrenic symptomatology in the absence of recent misuse (e.g. within the last month) a diagnosis of schizophrenia can be reliably made. In clinical practice, the picture is often less clear cut and a period of inpatient assessment may be necessary to clarify the diagnosis and tease out the relevant contributions of mental disorder and substance misuse to the clinical presentation. Assessment will be greatly helped by accessing a wide range of corroborative information sources including old clinical notes, general practitioners and relatives. Urine toxicology is essential but, as certain substances are undetectable 24–48 h after ingestion, samples for analysis need to been taken as soon possible if this window of diagnostic opportunity is not to be missed.

Service provision: whose patient anyway?

With expanding clinical recognition and research interest in dual diagnosis this question must surely strike a chord with many a generalist or addiction specialist having been faced with the challenge of managing patients with comorbidity. At best the patient receives either sequential treatment or concurrent parallel treatment by two separate services, and neither approach may be perfect (Drake *et al.* 1993; Crome 1999). At worst, the comorbid disorders may even be ignored (Hall & Farrell 1997). An ideal or standard approach for the management of dual diagnosis is not yet firmly established in the UK. There is as yet a limited number of studies on effective interventions and treatment outcome to guide service development (Miller 1994; Crome 1999).

In the USA, for example Drake *et al.* (1993) have described Continuous Treatment Teams and have identified nine emerging treatment principles of dual diagnosis treatment. These structural elements, which the authors claim underlie successful programmes, include: assertiveness, close monitoring, integration, comprehensiveness, stable living environment, flexibility and specialisation, stages of treatment (engagement, persuasion, active treatment and relapse prevention), longitudinal perspective and optimism! (Table 1.2).

Conclusion

Models of integrated inpatient treatment programmes have been described

Table 1.2 Principles of treatment of substance misuse in mentally ill patients.

ASSERTIVENESS	Outreach in the community
	Practical assistance with basic needs
	Working with family members
CLOSE MONITORING	Intensive supervision
	Voluntary and at times involuntary
INTEGRATION	Integrated treatment programmes in which the same clinician provides Mental Health and Substance Abuse in same setting
COMPREHENSIVENESS	Addresses living skills, relationships, vocational and interpersonal skills in addition to clinical treatments
STABLE LIVING ENVIRONMENT	Access to housing, support and companionship in the community
FLEXIBILITY AND SPECIALISATION	Successful administrators and clinicians modify previous beliefs, learn new skills and try new approaches empirically
STAGES OF TREATMENT	Treatment proceeds in stages: engagement, persuasion, active treatment and relapse prevention
LONGITUDINAL PERSPECTIVE	Recognises substance misuse and mental illness are chronic relapsing conditions and treatment occurs over years rather than episodically or during crisis
OPTIMISM	Encourages hope and counters demoralisation among patients, family and clinicians

Based on Drake *et al.* (1993).

(Minkoff 1989). However, it seems that with case management and assertive outreach dual diagnosis patients can be successfully engaged by community based services and at a relatively low cost (Drake & Noordsy 1994). It is even claimed that the expense involved in initiating such a programme need be little more than educating and supporting clinical staff while they develop the necessary skills for treating this group of patients. A central component therefore in many American treatment models is an integration for both mental illness treatment and addiction treatment which is delivered by the same team (Johnstone *et al.* 1999). Whether such models of specialist treatment services for dual diagnosed patients are appropriate or feasible in the UK and Europe is considered by Johnstone *et al.* (1999) who suggest that it may be preferable to try to develop ways of delivering integrated care within established sector community teams rather than trying to adopt the American model of distinct ultra-specialist dual diagnosis teams/services. Much of future developments in this area may depend on existing services, however, a number of authors (e.g. Johnson 1997; Crome 1999; Seivewright 1999) have described possible treatment models based on existing services. In a proposal to improve treatment for these patients, Hall and Farrell (1997) highlight the need to facilitate staff in both treatment settings to recognise and manage common comorbid conditions. This they suggest might modestly be achieved by increased awareness, use of screening techniques and by the sharing of skills and support between addiction and mental health services.

References

American Psychiatric Association (APA) (1994) Position statement on the need for improved training for treatment of patients with combined substance use and other psychiatric disorders. *American Journal of Psychiatry* **151** (5), 795–796.

Bryant, K.J., Rounsaville, B., Spitzer, R.L. & Williams, J.B. (1992) Reliability of dual diagnosis substance dependence and psychiatric disorders. *Journal of Mental and Nervous Disorder* **180**, 251–257.

Cantwell, R., Brewin, J., Glazebrook, C. *et al.* (1999) Prevalence of substance misuse in first episode psychosis. *British Journal of Psychiatry* **174**, 150–153.

Cohen, S.I. (1995) Overdiagnosis of schizophrenia: role of alcohol and drug misuse. *The Lancet* **346**, 1541–1542.

Crome, I. (1999) Substance misuse and psychiatric comorbidity: towards improved service provision. *Drugs: education, prevention and policy* **6** (2), 151–174.

Davidson, K.M. (1995) Diagnosis of depression in alcohol dependence: changes with drinking status. *British Journal of Psychiatry* **166**, 199–204.

Drake, R.E., Bartels, S.J., Teague, G.B., Noordsy, D.L. & Clarke, R.E. (1993) Treatment of substance abuse in severely mentally ill patients. *Journal of Nervous and Mental Disease* **181**, 606–611.

Drake, R.E. & Noordsy, D.L. (1994) Case management for people with coexisting severe mental disorder and substance use disorder. *Psychiatric Annals* **24**, 427–431.

El-Guebaly, N. (1990) Substance abuse and mental disorders: the dual diagnosis concept. *Canadian Journal of Psychiatry* **35**, 261–267.

El-Guebaly, N. (1995) Substance misuse disorders and mental illness: the relevance of comorbidity. *Canadian Journal of Psychiatry* **40**, 2–3.

Farrell, M., Howes, S., Taylor, C. *et al.* (1998) Substance misuse and psychiatric comorbidity: an overview of the OPCS National Psychiatric Morbidity Study. *Addictive Behaviours* **23** (6), 909–918.

Gossop, M., Marsden, J. & Steward, D. (1998) NTORS at one year: The National Treatment Outcome and Research Study. Department of Health, London.

Gupta, S., Hendricks, S., Kenkel, A.M., Bhatia, S.C. & Haffke, E.A. (1996) Relapse in schizophrenia: is there a relationship to substance misuse? *Schizophrenia Research* **20**, 153–156.

Hall, W. & Farrell, M. (1997) Comorbidity of mental disorders with substance misuse, *British Journal of Psychiatry* **171**, 4–5.

Johns, A. (1998) Substance misuse and offending. *Current Opinion in Psychiatry* **11**, 669–673.

Johnson, S. (1997) Dual diagnosis and severe mental illness and substance misuse: a case for specialist services? *British Journal of Psychiatry* **171**, 205–208.

Johnstone, E.C., Humphries, M.S., Lang, P.H., Lawrie, S.M. & Sandler, R. (1999) *Schizophrenia*. Cambridge University Press, Cambridge.

Khalsa, H.K., Shaner, A., Anglin, M.D. *et al.* (1991) Prevalence of substance abuse in a psychiatric evaluation unit. *Drug and Alcohol Dependence* **28**, 215–223.

Khantzian, E.J. (1985) The self-medication hypothesis of addiction disorders: focus on heroin and cocaine dependence. *American Journal of Psychiatry* **142**, 1259–1264.

Kosten, T.R. & Ziedonis, D.M. (1997) Substance misuse and schizophrenia, eds' introduction. *Schizophrenia Bulletin* **23** (2), 181–186.

Laurence, J. (1995) Mental hospitals are 'paradise for drug-pushers'. *The Times* 14 June, 6.

Lehman, A.F., Meyers, C.P. & Corty, E. (1989) Classification of patients with psychiatric and substance abuse syndromes. *Hospital and Community Psychiatry* **40** (10), 1019–1025.

McGuire, P.K., Jones, P., Harvey, I. *et al.* (1994) Cannabis and acute psychosis. *Schizophrenia Research* **13**, 161–168.

Menezes, P.R., Johnson, S., Thornicroft, G. *et al.* (1996) Drug and alcohol problems among individuals with severe mental illness in South London. *British Journal of Psychiatry* **168**, 612–619.

Miller, N.S. (1994) Prevalence and treatment models for addiction in psychiatric populations. *Psychiatric Annals* **24**, 399–406.

Minkoff, K. (1989) An integrated treatment model for dual diagnosis of psychosis and addiction. *Hospital and Community Psychiatry* **40**, 1031–1036.

Mueser, K.T., Bellack, A.S. & Blanchard, J.J. (1992) Comorbidity of schizophrenia and substance abuse: implications for treatment. *Journal of Consulting and Clinical Psychology* **60** (6), 845–856.

Mueser, K.T., Drake, R.E. & Wallach, M.E. (1998) Dual diagnosis: a review of etiological theories. *Addictive Behaviours* **23** (6), 717–734.

Neeleman, J. & Farrell, M. (1997) Suicide and substance misuse. *British Journal of Psychiatry* **175**, 303–304.

Negrete, J.C., Knapp, W.P., Douglas, D.E. & Smith, W.B. (1986) Cannabis affects the severity of schizophrenic symptoms: results of a clinical survey. *Psychological Medicine* **16**, 515–520.

Office of Population Censuses and Surveys (1994) Survey of psychiatric morbidity in Great Britain. *Bulletin No. 1 Office of National Statistics*. HMSO, London.

Oyefeso, A., Ghodse, H., Clancy, C. & Corkey, J. (1999) Suicide among drug addicts in the UK. *British Journal of Psychiatry* **175**, 277–282.

Poole, R. & Brabbins, C. (1996) Drug induced psychosis. *British Journal of Psychiatry* **168**, 135–138.

Pristach, C.A. & Smith, C.M. (1990) Medication compliance and substance abuse among schizophrenic patients. *Hospital and Community Psychiatry* **41**, 1345–1348.

Regier, D.A., Farmer, M.E., Rae, D.S. *et al.* (1990) Comorbidity of mental disorders with alcohol and other drug abuse: results from the Epidemiological Catchment Area (ECA) Study. *Journal of the American Medical Association* **264**, 2511–2518.

Rosenthal, R.N. & Miner, C.R. (1997) Differential diagnosis of substance-induced psychosis and schizophrenia in patients with substance use disorders. *Schizophrenia Bulletin* **23** (2), 187–193.

Rostad, P. & Checinski, K. (1996) Dual diagnosis: facing the challenge. *The Care of People with Dual Diagnosis of Mental Illness and Substance Misuse*. Wynne Howard Publishing, Surrey.

Rounsaville, B.J., Weissman, M.M., Crits-Christopher, K., Wilber, C. & Kleber, H. (1982) Diagnosis and symptoms of depression in opiate addicts: course and relation to treatment outcome. *Archives of General Psychiatry* **39**, 151–156.

Scott, H., Johnson, S., Menezes, P.R., Thornicroft, G., Marshall, J., Bindman, J., Bebbington, P. & Kuipers, E. (1999) Substance misuse and risk of aggression and offending among the severely mental ill. *British Journal of Psychiatry* **172**, 345–350.

Seivewright, S., ed. (1999) *Dual Diagnosis–Drug Misuse and Psychiatric Disorder*. In: *Community Treatment of Drug Misuse: More than methadone*. Cambridge University Press, Cambridge, pp. 190–203.

Shaffer, D., Gould, M.S., Fisher, P. *et al.* (1996) Psychiatric diagnosis in child and adolescent suicide. *Archives of General Psychiatry* **53**, 339–348.

Smith, J. & Hucker, S. (1994) Schizophrenia and substance abuse. *British Journal of Psychiatry* **165**, 13–21.

Sokolshi, K.N., Cummings, J.L., Abrams, B.I., DeMet, E.M., Kalz, L.S. & Costa, J.F. (1994) Effects of substance misuse on hallucination rates and treatment response in chronic psychiatric patients. *Journal of Clinical Psychiatry* **55**, 380–387.

Weiss, R.D., Mirin, S.M. & Griffin, M.L. (1992) Methodological considerations in the diagnosis of coexisting psychiatric disorders in substance abusers. *British Journal of Addiction* **87**, 179–187.

Williams, H. (1998) Dual diagnosis: fact or fiction for the practising clinician? *Irish Journal of Psychological Medicine* **15**, 3–5.

Williams, R. & Cohen, J. (2000) Substance use and misuse in psychiatric wards: a model task for clinical governance? *Psychiatric Bulletin* **24**, 43–46.

Wu, L., Kouzis, A.C. & Leaf, P.J. (1999) Influence of comorbid alcohol and psychiatric disorders on utilisation of mental health services in the national comorbidity study. *American Journal of Psychiatry* **156** (8), 1230–1236.

2: Substance Use and Dual Diagnosis: Concepts, Theories and Models

G. Hussein Rassool

Introduction

Using psychoactive substances has been and remains a universal phenomenon across all strata of society. It seems inevitable that all society will continue to be exposed to a myriad of drugs in the future. In the twentieth century, there was no dovetailing of interest in the use of psychoactive substances and plants. Psychoactive substances are substances that have an effect on the central nervous system in altering mood, cognitive process and behaviour. The range of drug varies from the misuse of tranquillisers, barbiturates, heroin, stimulants such as amphetamines and cocaine and its derivatives to cannabis and hallucinogens. The 'health-damaging' consumption of recreational, prescribed and illicit psychoactive substances worldwide has caused a host of social, behavioural, psychological and physical problems.

The medicinal use of psychoactive substances in both traditional and complementary therapies has profound therapeutic benefits that enable people to offset physical or psychological pathology, limit disability and to maintain their function more normally. The majority of adult populations of the Northern hemisphere use alcohol as a social lubricant, to relieve tension and anxiety or to facilitate social intercourse. Non-prescription, prescription and over-the-counter drugs are mainly used for similar purposes. However, an increasingly large segment of the population are misusing psychoactive drugs, licit and illicit, with physical, psychological, social, and/or legal consequences. Some individuals who have become acquainted with psychoactive substances through legitimate medical use are engaging in self-medication for the relief of a particular set of symptoms or to counterbalance the effects of other psychoactive substances.

The aims of this chapter are to provide an overview of the global drug scenes and examine the key concepts related to addiction and dependence. The drug experience, patterns of substance use and misuse, how people take drugs and theories and models of substance and dual diagnosis are presented.

Global drug scenes

The United Nations Office for Drug Control and Prevention (ODCCP 2000a) estimates that some 180 million people worldwide used illicit drugs in the 1990s. This includes 144 million for cannabis; 29 million for cocaine and 13.5 million for opiates (mainly heroin). The trend in the use of illicit drugs shows a stabilisation of opiates in Western Europe, and a decline of cocaine consumption in the United States. However, the amphetamine-type stimulants (ATS) began to show signs of stabilisation in some Western European countries towards the end of the decade but there is substantial growth in East and South-East Asia (ODCCP 2000a). During the 1990s, at least 134 countries and territories were faced with a drug misuse problem, with three-quarters of all countries reporting the use of illicit heroin and two-thirds misuse of cocaine (ODCCP 2000b). According to the World Health Organization (WHO 1998), there are over one billion smokers across the world resulting in 4 million deaths a year. There is an upward trend in tobacco smoking in Third World countries and in Eastern Europe. Alcohol-related diseases and injuries account for 3–4% of the annual global figure and there are around 750 000 alcohol-related deaths each year. Alcohol is a significant factor in hospital admissions, road traffic deaths, industrial accidents, accidental drownings, homicide and suicide (WHO 1998).

In the United Kingdom (UK) there are approximately 13 million adults who smoke. This population smokes more cigarettes than the European average, costing the National Health Service up to £1.7 billion each year. Currently, more than 120 000 people die each year in the UK from tobacco smoking (Department of Health 1998). It is estimated that the annual prevalence rate of alcohol dependence in private households is 75 per thousand among men aged 16–24 years and 21 per thousand of the population among women in the same age group. In Great Britain, there were 168 000 casualties in traffic accidents involving illegal alcohol levels (5% of all traffic accident casualties) (Statistical Bulletin 1999). In the UK, it is estimated that 6% of the population, around 3 million people, take at least one illegal drug in any one year (Tackling Drugs Together 1995). In 1998, among those aged 16–24 years in England and Wales, 29% had used drugs in the previous year and 19% in the previous month. Twenty-seven per cent (27%) reported having used cannabis in the previous year, 10% amphetamines, 5% ecstasy, 5% poppers, 3% cocaine and fewer than 0.5% crack or heroin. Although the figure among those aged 16–24 who had used drugs in the previous year was the same as previous years, cocaine was the only drug showing a significant increase from 1% in 1994 to 3% in 1998 (Statistical Bulletin 2000).

Key concepts related to addiction

Drug and drug misuse

What constitutes a drug (food is considered a drug) depends on various factors as the concept is heavily influenced by the sociocultural context and purpose of its use. The therapeutic use of 'drug' means a pharmacological preparation used in the prevention, diagnosis and treatment of an abnormal or pathological condition whereas the non-therapeutic use of drugs is commonly referred to the use of illegal or socially disapproved substances (Rassool 1998). However, drugs can be either therapeutic or non-therapeutic or both. Throughout history there has been often an arbitrary way in which society has defined a 'drug' and the change in connotation is regarded as a product of social custom and law, both of which change over time (Smith 1970). According to the World Health Organization (1981), a drug is defined as

> 'Any chemicals entity or mixture of entities, other than those required for the maintenance of normal health (like food), the administration of which alters biological function and possibly structure.'

Despite the broadness of the concept, which limits its use for clinical and for certain practical purposes, it provides some perspective into its ubiquitous nature. A drug, in the broadest sense, is a chemical substance that has an effect on bodily systems and behaviour. The term drug misuse may be seen as the use of drugs in a socially unacceptable way that is harmful or hazardous to the individual or others (World Health Organization 1981; ISDD 1996; Royal College of Psychiatrists & Royal College of Physicians 2000). It can also be taken to mean the use of a drug which carries implications of illegality or harmfulness and used without medical approval. The Royal College of Psychiatrists (1987) defines drug misuse as

> '. . . Any taking of a drug which harms or threatens to harm the physical or mental health or social well-being of an individual, or other individuals, or of society at large, or which is illegal.'

This broad definition encompasses the misuse of alcohol, prescribed drugs such as temazepan or diazepam and illicit drugs such as heroin or cocaine. The World Health Organization recommends the use of the following terms:

- *Unsanctioned use*: a drug that is not approved of by society
- *Hazardous use*: a drug leading to harm or dysfunction
- *Dysfunctional use*: a drug leading to impaired psychological or social functioning
- *Harmful use*: a drug that is known to cause tissue damage or psychiatric disorders.

Substance abuse and dependence

The terms substance use and abuse are difficult concepts to define precisely but the operational use of these concepts is heavily dependent on particular culture, ideology, aetiology and clinical practice (Rassool 1998). Substance use is defined as the ingestion of a substance that is used for therapeutic purpose or as prescribed by medical practitioners. Substance misuse is the result of a psychoactive substance being consumed in a way that it was not intended for and which causes physical, social and psychological harm. It is also used to represent the pattern of use: experimental, recreational and dependent. The term substance abuse, often associated with addiction and dependence, is considered to be value-laden and has limited use in the addiction literature in the United Kingdom. In the United States, practitioners prefer the term substance abuse for problems resulting from the use of alcohol or other mood-altering drugs and use addictive disorders when the problems have escalated to dependency (Sullivan 1995). According to Fleming *et al.* (1996), substance abuse is used in two different ways: a diagnostic term—'it is intermittent impaired control of substance use and represents a stage in the spectrum of substance use disorders' and colloquially, 'it describes drug use that violates social standards or causes self-harm'. Whether a substance is used or abused depends very much on the social and cultural context, the individual perspective, the pattern and mode of consumption and the perception of the observer. Abuse, according to DSM-IV (APA 1994), requires that one or more criteria occur at any time during the same 12-month period. The DSM-IV criteria for abuse is briefly presented in Table 2.1.

The concept of drug *dependence* is associated with the World Health Organization (WHO 1969) and has the advantage of a universal definition. The WHO defined drug dependence as

> 'a state, psychic and sometimes also physical, resulting from the interaction between a living organism and a drug, characterised by behavioural and other responses that always include a compulsion to take the drug on a continuous or periodic basis in order to experience its physical effects, and sometimes to avoid the discomfort of its absence. Tolerance may or may not be present. A person may be dependent on more than one drug.' (p.14)

This comprehensive definition has been widely accepted and highlights the core features of dependence such as tolerance, psychological and physical dependence. These concepts need further explanations and are examined

Table 2.1 DSM-IV diagnostic criteria for substance abuse

A. A maladaptive pattern of substance use leading to clinically significant impairment or distress, as manifested by one or more of the following occurring during the same 12-month period:

Recurrent substance use resulting in a failure to fulfil major role obligations at work, school, or home (e.g. repeated absences or poor work performance related to substance use; substance-related absences, suspensions, or expulsions from school; neglect of children and household)

Recurrent substance use in situations in which it is physically hazardous (e.g. driving an automobile or operating a machine when impaired by substance use)

Recurrent substance-related legal problems (e.g. arrests for substance-related disorderly conduct)

Continued substance use despite having persistent or recurrent effects or interpersonal problems caused or exacerbated by the effects of the susbtance.

B. The above symptoms have not met the criteria for substance dependence for this class of substance.

Source: APA (1994)

Table 2.2 DSM-IV diagnostic criteria for substance dependence

A maladaptive pattern of substance use leading to clinically significant impairment or distress, as manifested by three or more of the following occurring during the same 12-month period:
1. Tolerance, as defined by either of the following:
   Need for markedly increased amounts of the substance to achieve intoxication or desired effect
   Markedly diminished effect of continued use of the same amount of the substance
2. Withdrawal, as manifested by either of the following:
   The characteristic withdrawal syndrome for the substance
   The same (or a closely related) substance is taken to relieve or avoid withdrawal symptoms
3. The substance is often taken in larger amounts or over a long period than was intended.
4. A persistent desire or unsuccessful efforts to cut down or control substance use
5. A great deal of time is spent in activities necessary to obtain the substance (e.g. visiting multiple doctors or driving long distances), use of substance (e.g. chain-smoking), or recover from its effects
6. Important social, occupational, or recreational activities are given up or reduced because of substance use
7. The substance use is continued despite knowledge of having a persistent or recurrent physical or psychological problem that is likely to have been caused or exacerbated by the substance (e.g. current cocaine-induced depression, or continued drinking despite recognition that an ulcer was made worse by alcohol consumption)

Source: APA (1994)

in the next section. Dependence, according to DSM-IV (APA 1994), requires that three out of seven criteria occurring at any time in the same 12-month period. The DSM-IV criteria for dependence are briefly presented in Table 2.2. Dependence is also seen as comparable to addiction as 'the user has adapted physically and/or psychologically to the presence of the drug and would suffer if it is withdrawn' (RCP 2000).

Psychological and physical dependence

Tolerance

Tolerance is a behavioural state and refers to the way the body usually adapts to the repeated presence of a drug. Higher quantities or doses of the psychoactive substance are required to reproduce the desired or similar cognitive, affective or behavioural effects. Tolerance may develop rapidly in the case of LSD or slowly in the case of alcohol or opiates. The drug must be taken on a regular basis and in adequate quantities for tolerance to occur. For example, amphetamines can produce considerable tolerance and strong psychological dependence with little or no physical dependence, and cocaine can produce psychological dependence without tolerance or physical dependence. Furthermore, in certain medical applications, morphine has been reported to produce tolerance and physical dependence without a significant psychological component. Tolerance can be subdivided into: *phar-*

macodynamic tolerance, when higher doses of the drug are needed to produce the desired response or effect; *metabolic tolerance,* when there is an increase in capacity to metabolise a drug; and *cross tolerance,* when one is tolerant to one drug, there is also tolerance to other drugs of the same type or classification (Schuckit 1995).

Psychological dependence

Psychological dependence can be described as a compulsion or a craving to continue to take the drug because of the need for stimulation, or because it relieves anxiety or depression. Psychological dependence is recognised as the most widespread and the most important (ISDD 1996). This kind of dependence is not only attributed to the use of psychoactive drugs but also to food, sex, gambling, relationships or physical activities.

Physical dependence

Physical dependence is a state of bodily adaptation to the presence of a particular psychoactive drug. This manifests itself in physical disturbances or withdrawal symptoms following cessation of use. The withdrawal symptoms depend on the type or category of drug. For example, for nicotine, the physiological withdrawal symptoms may be relatively slight. In other dependence-inducing psychoactive substances such as opiates and depressants, the withdrawal experience can range from mild to severe. The withdrawal from alcohol for instance can cause hallucinations or epileptic fits and may be life-threatening. In the case of heroin withdrawal, physical symptoms such as diarrhoea, running nose and cramps, etc. are present. Physical withdrawal syndromes are not, however, the essence of dependence. It is possible to have dependence without withdrawal and withdrawal without dependence (Royal College of Psychiatrists 1987). However, it is argued that many of the supposed signs of physical dependence are sometimes psychosomatic reactions triggered off not by the chemical properties of psychoactive drugs but by the user's fears, beliefs and fantasies about what withdrawal entails (Plant 1987).

The dependence syndrome

The original framework of the dependence syndrome referred specifically to alcohol dependence but this has been expanded to include other psychoactive substances. According to Edwards and Gross (1976), there are seven components of the syndrome:

(1) Increased tolerance to the drug.
(2) Repeated withdrawal symptoms.
(3) Compulsion to use the drug (psychological state known as craving).
(4) Salience of drug-seeking behaviour (obtaining and using the drug become more important in the person's life).

17

(5) Relief or avoidance of withdrawal symptoms (the regular use of the drug to relieve withdrawal symptoms).

(6) Narrowing of the repertoire of drug taking (pattern of drinking may become an everyday activity).

(7) Rapid reinstatement after abstinence.

The dependence syndrome, derived from the disease's biological and behavioural models, has provided a common language for academics and clinicians to talk about the same phenomena. According to Drummond (1991), the dependent concept has helped in sharpening up diagnostic precision, predicting treatment needs and has also provided a means of making experiences intelligible to the problem drinker or problem drug user. However, the concept has been criticised by both Narcotics Anonymous advocates and cognitive behavioural psychologists as being closed related to the disease model and physiological perspectives (Keene 1997).

Addictive behaviour

Addictive behaviour is a complex dynamic behaviour pattern having psychological, physical, social and behavioural components. Miller (1990) states that addictive behaviour can be construed by the presence of three behavioural characteristics:

(1) lifestyle being focused around obtaining the substance;

(2) the compulsion to use; and

(3) the presence of relapse.

This narrow perspective is more appropriate when referring only to pharmacological substances. According to Marlatt *et al.* (1988) addictive behaviour is defined as

> 'a repetitive habit pattern that increases the risk of diseases and/or associated personal or social problems. The individual usually has a loss of control, immediate gratification with delayed, deleterious effects, and experiences relapses when trying to quit.'

This wide-ranging definition seems to be quite vague and fails to explain the potential contributory factors in the development of this kind of behaviour. Addictive behaviour includes the misuse of psychoactive substances and activities leading to excessive behavioural patterns. Individuals who have problems with excessive behaviours such as eating, drinking, drug use, gambling and sexuality present similar descriptions of the phenomenology of their disorders (Wallace 1977; Cummings *et al.* 1980; Stall & Biernacki 1981; Orford 1985). This entails the classification of both pharmacological and non-pharmacological addictions under the more inclusive diagnostic category of addictive behaviour (Marks 1990; Ghodse 1995).

Problem drug users

The Advisory Council on the Misuse of Drugs (ACMD) report on 'Treatment and Rehabilitation' (ACMD 1982) defines problem drug user as

'. . . any person who experiences social, psychological, physical or legal problems related to intoxication and\or regular excessive consumption and\or dependence as a consequence of his own use of drugs or other chemical substances.'

This definition was widened to include any form of drug misuse that involves, or may lead to, sharing of injecting equipment (ACMD 1988). The above definition focuses on the needs and problems of the individual and places less emphasis on the substance-oriented approach. It is a holistic definition in acknowledging that the problem drug user has social, psychological, physical and legal needs and the definition could be expanded to incorporate the spiritual needs of the individual of the problem drug user or problem drinker. A more recent complementary definition (RCP 2000) indicates that 'either the pattern of drug taking, or the route of administration is causing significant physical, psychological or social problems for the user and generally implies greater harm than drug misuse'. However, the definition seems to convey that the difference between drug misuse and problem drug use is related to the degree of harm caused by the drug.

Drug experience

It is acknowledged that the effect of a psychoactive substance or 'drug experience' on a given individual will depend on several other factors beside the pharmacological properties of the drug. The gamut of drug experience involves interrelated sets of non-pharmacological and pharmacological factors. These include pharmacological factors, personality of the individual and the context or setting (Ghodse 1989). The pharmacological factors include the chemical properties or type of drug used. Different drugs have different mode of action on the body due to its pharmacological properties, the drug dosage and the route of administration. In addition, the effects or actions of a psychoactive drug are influenced by the personal characteristics of the drug user. These characteristics include factors such as the person's biological makeup, personality, gender, age and drug tolerance (Rassool 1998). For instance, some individuals may develop a toxic reaction to a single cup of coffee or the normally insignificant elevation of heart rate caused by cannabis can be painful for those suffering from angina pectoris, whereas glaucoma patients may find cannabis beneficial but a few cups of coffee may aggravate their conditions (ISDD 1996). In addition, the knowledge, attitude and expectations (psychological set) about a drug will have an influence on the 'drug experience'. For example, if an individual believes or expects—as a self-fulfilling prophecy—that a particular substance will produce a certain effect, the desired effect may be experienced. The last set of factors is the setting or context in which a drug is used. This includes the physical environment where the drug is used, the cultural influences of the community where the drug is consumed, the laws related to drug use and the context in which a drug is used.

All the three interrelated factors, pharmacological properties, individual

19

differences and context of use influence the individual experiences of drug taking. It is stated that 'it is necessary to see the drug–brain interaction not as a simple chemical event but as a matter of considerable complexity involving the drug, the particular person, and the messages and teachings which come from the environment and which powerfully influence the nature and meaning of the drug experience' (Royal College of Psychiatrists 1987).

Patterns of substance use and misuse

The patterns of drug or alcohol use and misuse for some individuals sometimes vary over a period of time. The patterns of substance misuse are often described as *experimental, recreational* and *problematic*.

Experimental users

Experimental users are described as those who have used drugs, legal or illicit, on a few occasions. By definition, anyone's initial use of a drug, alcohol or smoking tobacco is experimental (Rassool 1998). The main motivation for experimental drug or alcohol use includes curiosity, anticipation of effects and availability. This usually forms part of the desire among adolescents to experiment and try risky new experiences. There is no pattern in the use of psychoactive substances but the choice of the drug misused is indiscriminate. The choice of drug use depends on factors such as availability, social marketing, reputation of the drug, subculture, fashion and peer-group influence. Experimental use of illicit psychoactive substances is usually a short-lived experience and the majority of people may confine their consumption to drugs that are socially acceptable. Experimental users, however, are in the highest category of risk for infections (if injecting), medical complications or overdose due to the indiscriminate use of adulterated psychoactive substances. It has been suggested that the likelihood of 'their future significant engagement with, or disengagement from, further drug use has not yet been firmly determined' (RCP 2000).

Recreational users

Experimental users may or may not become recreational users of illicit psychoactive substances. The term 'recreational' refers to a form of substance use in which pleasure and relaxation are the prime motivations. There is a strict adherence to the pattern of use so that the drug is only used on certain occasions such as weekends and is less likely on consecutive days. There is usually a preference for a particular drug (drug of choice), once an individual has learned how to use it and appreciate its effects. Drug or alcohol use is one aspect of the user's life and tends to complement social and recreational activities. There are usually no adverse medical or social consequences as a result of recreational use such as in the case of controlled drinking.

Dependent users

By definition, a dependent user has progressed to regular and problematic use of a psychoactive drug or becoming a poly-drug user. There is the presence of psychological and/or physical dependence and therefore such use is distinguished from experimental and recreational use. The pattern of use is more frequent and regular but less controlled. The process in obtaining the drug is more important to the user than the quality of experience. This tends to displace rather than complement social activities. Injecting drugs is common, and frequent use creates problems of intoxication, infections if sharing needles and syringes, and other medical complications. Personal, social, psychological and legal problems may be present in this group.

Routes of drug administration

The common routes of taking drug are orally, or by smoking, inhalation and injection. According to Rawaf and Schifano (2000) there is a trend in European youth culture that only the molecules which can be snorted, inhaled or ingested are considered acceptable. The route of administration is very important in the speed of influencing the physical and psychological effects of the drug.

Oral

The oral route (swallowing) is the most popular method of drug administration although effectively the slowest route because of the slow absorption of the drug into the bloodstream. It is stated that unlike the injection or inhalation routes, there is little stigma associated with taking drugs orally either in pills or in the form of beverages containing alcohol or caffeine (Schilit & Lisansky Gomberg 1991, p.17).

Injecting

The methods of drug injecting include intramuscularly or subcutaneously/intravenously. Injection of drugs is less widespread than other routes of drug administration but also the most hazardous. The major dangers of injecting are risk of overdose because of the concentrated effect of this method. There is also the risk of infection from non-sterile injection methods including hepatitis B and HIV infections, abscesses, gangrene, and thromboses. The onset of the effects of the drug is rapid when it is administered intravenously and is a major reason why drugs are often self-administered by injecting. Drugs that are mainly injected include heroin, cocaine, amphetamines and some hypno-sedatives. However, injecting heroin in Southern Europe is not considered fashionable any longer (Rawaf & Schifano 2000).

Inhalation

The inhalation route (sniff) is also used to self-administer drugs. Absorption of the drug is through the mucous membrane of the nose and mouth. The types of drugs that are inhaled include cocaine, tobacco in the form of snuff and volatile substances and solvents. Inhalation may also produce rapid absorption and response as in the case of crack cocaine.

Smoking

Smoking is also a very effective route as the drug is inhaled as in the case of tobacco or heroin smoking (chasing the dragon). Cannabis or marijuana, usually mixed with tobacco, is also smoked in the form of a 'joint'.

Theoretical models of substance misuse

Many models and theories have peen put forth to explain why people use or misuse psychoactive substances and about the causes of substance misuse. The theories provide explanations for the initiation into substance misuse or for why individuals begin to use drugs and the process of addiction. Some theories explain both initial and continuing use of drugs (Addiction Research Foundation 1986). However, the reason why people start using drugs may not be the same reason why they continue to use drugs. It will become apparent that no single theory is sufficient to explain substance use and misuse *per se*, and that that a range of 'risk factors' has to be considered. Most of the studies are retrospective in design and more research has been conducted in relation to alcohol rather than any other substances.

Disease theory

The disease concept of alcoholism was initially proposed by Jellinek (1960). This model views substance misuse as a progressive incurable disorder and the cause of the disease is firmly attributed to the genetic/biological makeup of the individual (Jellinek 1960; Valliant 1983). According to the disease theory of alcoholism, once a drink is taken, craving is increased and the physical demand for alcohol overrides any cognitive or voluntary control (Jellinek 1960). The notion that alcohol in the bloodstream itself precipitates involuntary drinking has been refuted by experimental research. This disease approach also implies the adoption of the sick-role by the substance misusers and the individuals are expected to be treated as having a 'disease'. The treatment approach also implies that recovery from drug or alcohol misuse can only be sustained through the goal of total abstinence within the self-help group movements such as 'AA', 'NA' and 'GA' (Alcoholics Anonymous, Narcotics Anonymous, Gamblers Anonymous). The disease concept of addictive behaviour is incorporated in the philosophy underpinning the approaches of NA or AA in the adoption of the Minnesota Model (Cook 1988). However, the disease model of substance use reduces the scope of analysis to features that are physiological in origin and isolates the importance of the interrelationship of both psychological and sociocultural factors in the maintenance of substance use behaviour.

Genetic theory

A number of studies have suggested that substance misuse is the result of genetic or induced biological abnormality of a physiological, structural or chemical nature. There is strong evidence that early onset alcoholism is genetically determined (Cloninger 1987; Blum *et al.* 1990; Pickens *et al.* 1991). Problem drinkers have a 50% chance of having at least one member of their family becoming dependent on alcohol and there is a 90% chance of two or more family members being so dependent (Miller 1991). In adoption studies, children whose adopted parents were dependent on alcohol, were more likely themselves to develop a problem with alcohol, though their biological parents were not dependent on alcohol (Miller 1991). However, the findings of the Copenhagen study (Goodwin *et al.* 1977), which is the best on methodological grounds to date, showed that there was a fourfold increase in the incidence of alcoholism among male adoptees who were removed from their alcoholic parents soon after birth. In a study of pairs of twins by Tsuang *et al.* (1996), the findings suggest the likelihood of developing a dependence on opiates or stimulants was influenced by genetic factors than by shared environmental factors. Some people may experience a less intense reaction to alcohol and such vulnerable individuals drink more before feeling intoxicated. It also appears that a genetic predisposition may also protect some individuals who have a genetically based metabolic sensitivity to indulging in psychoactive substances, such as alcohol (Wolf 1972). The available data so far indicate that dependence on alcohol is a genetically influenced disorder with a rate of heritability similar to that expected for diabetes or peptic ulcers (Schuckit 1995).

There are different methodologies used in several studies (mainly alcohol studies) such as face-to-face interviews, records such as hospitalisation and arrests, and the use of different operational definitions of alcoholism. This may have implications in comparing and confirming the different findings, especially in adoption and twin studies. However, the review by Adityanjee and Murray (1991) of twin studies of alcoholism and normal drinking looks at a number of studies in a similar culture and racial group that indicate that alcoholism tends to run in families but acknowledge that no one is clear about what it is that may or may not be transmitted through genetic inheritance.

Psychological theories

There are a number of psychological theories that attempt to explain the causation of drug and alcohol dependent behaviour. A brief overview of selected theories is presented here.

Psychoanalytic theory is derived from the work of Freud based on the components of the self and their functioning during the stages of psychosexual development. However, Freud made little reference to alcoholism in his published work but did suggest that the consumption of alcohol provided relief from the conflict generated by oral fixation, or repressed homosexuality. According to the psychoanalytic theory, adaptive behaviour requires the harmonious functioning of the id, ego and super ego (the self). These components change during the stages of psychosexual development. Alcoholism and other pathological conditions are attributed to the conflicts in these stages of development, resulting in the destructive interactions among the three components of the self. The aetiology of alcohol or drug dependence is assumed to develop from sensual satisfaction (avoidance of pain or anxiety), conflict among the id, ego and super ego and fixation in the infantile past (Allen 1996). In order to avoid pain or anxiety, alcohol intoxication is assumed to provide this relief.

Mental defence mechanisms seem to operate in the case of conflicts among the components of the self. Denial, repression, projection and displacement can be seen as part of the behavioural repertoire. The use of alcohol or a drug (smoking) is related to the 'fixation' at the oral stage of development. According to Treece and Khantzian (1986), there are certain pychodynamic characteristics observed in substance-dependent individuals. These include problems in affect management, narcissism, object relations, judgement and self-care. These problems may predispose individuals to drug dependence because they are the basis of anxieties or distresses that are relieved by taking psychoactive substances. Dependency involves the gradual incorporation of the drug effects and the user's experienced need into the defensive structure building activity of the ego itself (Treece & Khantzian 1986). There are major methodological problems with psychoanalytic studies and no empirical evidence has been found to support this theory.

In behavioural theories, the use of psychoactive substances is viewed as an acquired behaviour, a response that is learned through the process of classical conditioning (Pavlovian conditioning), operant conditioning (Skinner) and social learning. In classical conditioning, dependence is in part acquired through the process of associative learning. That is, the desire to use drugs may be the result of specific factors associated with the use of a particular substance. The maintenance of drug-taking behaviour is the result of past associations with drug-taking environment or situation. Wikler (1948, 1961) first suggested the significant role played by classical conditioning in the development of the motivation to use drugs. However, the theory of classical conditioning does not make provision for individual differences (genetic factors), social factors or the expectations of drug effects. In operant conditioning learning occurs when the response or behaviour is followed by reinforcement. Reinforcements strengthen behaviour and may be positive (rewarding behaviour) or negative (avoidance of an unpleasant experience). The role of positive reinforcement in the use of psychoactive substances can be explained by the fact that drugs can cause pleasurable sensations. The more pleasure or in some cases fear of withdrawal reinforces the continued use of the substance.

Social learning theory (or cognitive social learning) provides an explanation of how behaviour (adaptive or maladaptive) is formed and maintained through the process of positive and negative reinforcement. Behaviour is assumed to be also influenced by role modelling and the need to conform. Studies (Becker 1966; Bandura 1977; Collins & Marlatt 1981; Barnes 1990) have demonstrated that modelling affects drinking behaviour. For example, how an individual's consumption of alcohol will vary to match that of a drinking partner. Their findings indicate that heavy drinking males seem to exhibit the strongest response to a heavy drinking model of the same sex. In effect, patterns of behaviour and attitudes can also be acquired through observation of social models without any reinforcement of overt behaviour. In the cognitive social learning theory, in order to understand the effects of alcohol or drugs, cognitive processes must be considered in relation to other factors. In addition, there is also an interrelationship between personal (expectations, beliefs, cognitions) and environmental factors (context, social setting). That is, an individual's prior experience with alcohol or drugs and the social setting in which drinking or drug taking occurs must be considered.

Other cognitive theories or models include the tension-reduction theory, self-awareness model and the expectancy theory. The tension-reduction theory is based on the notion that individuals drink in order to reduce tension or anxiety. The drinking of alcohol or taking drugs becomes the reinforcer because it produces a reduction in tension (Cappell & Greeley 1987). The self-awareness model (Hull 1981) attempts to understand the cause and effects of psychoactive substances in terms of disinhibiting social behaviour by reducing an individual's level of self-awareness. The expectancy theory seeks to explain the role of cognitive factors in the initiation of substance use and the maintenance of drug-taking behaviour despite the consequences. (Stacy et al. 1990). This theory focuses on beliefs about psychoactive substance that develop at an early age. 'Outcome expectancy' may link drug or alcohol use with a specific incoming situation. Studies amongst adolescents show that expectations predicted drinking behaviour more accurately than social background and demographic variables (ethnicity, religious affiliation, parental attitudes) and that subjects believed that alcohol would improve their cognitive and motor functioning (Christiansen & Goldman 1983). Orford (1985) proposes a theory of 'Excessive Appetites' within the context of social learning paradigm. He develops a theory of addiction and maintains that the degree of an individual's involvement with 'appetitive activities' has multiple interacting determinants. These include biological, personality, social and ecological determinants.

Within the framework of psychological theories, personality theory stresses the importance of personal traits and characteristics in the formation and maintenance of dependence. Traits such as hyperactivity, sensation-seeking, antisocial behaviour and impulsivity have been found to be associated with substance misuse (Sher *et al*. 1991). According to Ghodse (1995) while 'there is an epidemiological association between drug misuse and personality disorder, no deductions can be made about causality as most studies have compared drug-dependent with non-dependent individuals' (p. 20). He asserted that there might be personality traits that change the likelihood of an individual becoming dependent on drugs.

Sociocultural theories

Sociocultural theories include a number of subtheories such as *systems theory, family interaction theory, anthropological theory, economic theory, gateway theory* and *availability theory*. For a discussion of these theories see National Institute on Alcohol Abuse and Alcoholism and Center for Substance Abuse Prevention (1993). In the systems theory, behaviour is determined and maintained by the ongoing demands of interpersonal systems in which an individual interacts. The aetiology is based on behaviour observed in family contexts such as behaviour resulting from the interactions between relevant significant others. Steinglass's (1987) work supports the idea of alcoholism as a 'family disease' or 'family disorder'. In the family interaction theory, the most significant aetiological factor is probably parental deficits that occur as a product of parental alcoholism. These deficits may include parental absence, family tension, rejection, emotional distancing and parental alienation. There is also some evidence to suggest that alcohol may serve as an adaptive function in a marital relationship by facilitation of interaction (Jacob & Leonard 1988).

The availability theory suggests that the greater the availability of alcohol or other psychoactive substances, the greater the prevalence and severity of substance use problems in society. According to Ghodse (1995), the availability of the drug is a prerequisite for misuse and dependence and the rapid transport systems of the modern world ensure that drugs or alcohol are obtainable everywhere. Influences such as availability of drugs, relative cost, social pressures, legal sanctions and marketing practices are the best predictors of the development of dependence (Henningfield *et al*. 1991). Other sociocultural factors that may have an influence on the choice between drug and alcohol use and misuse include gender, age, occupation, social class, ethno-cultural background, subcultures, alienated groups, family dysfunction and religious affiliation.

Bio-psychosocial theory

There have been several attempts to amalgamate the biological, psychological and sociological theories of drug and alcohol dependence into a mega theory—the bio-psychosocial perspective (Galizio & Maisto 1985; Kumpter *et al.* 1990; Wallace 1990). The bio-psychosocial model takes into consideration a broad range of factors which interact, resulting in addiction. Thus, drug and alcohol dependence are viewed as the result of multifactorial causation rather than having unidimensional cause. The bio-psychosocial 'vulnerability model' of Kumpter *et al.* includes biological factors (genetic inheritance, physiological differences), psychosocial and environmental factors (family, community, peer or social pressure). The model views these factors 'as temporarily ordered in its interactions', so leading to addiction. Whether the goal is prevention, treatment or research, health care professionals can understand the individuals from a holistic perspective.

Theories and models of dual diagnosis

There are a variety of models and theories that hypothesize why severe mentally ill patients are vulnerable in the misuse of psychoactive substances. These models, according to Mueser *et al.* (1998) can generally be divided into two types: the *psychosocial risk factor* models and the *supersensitivity* model. The psychosocial risk models include the self-medication hypothesis, the alleviation of dysphoria model and the multiple risk factor model.

Psychosocial risk factor models

Self-medication hypothesis

A model of self-medication as an aetiological factor in substance misuse was proposed by Khantzian (1985, 1997), on the basis of psychodynamic/psychiatric diagnostic findings and clinical observations. Self-medication refers to the motivation of patients to seek a specific drug for relief of a particular set of symptoms. Khantzian (1985, 1997) suggested that individuals misuse psychoactive substances adaptively to cope with painful affective states and related psychiatric disorders which may predispose them to addictive behaviours. He stated that potential addicts, selection of specific psychoactive substances are not chosen at random but for their unique effects. Khantzian (1997) argues that an opiate user may self-medicate with, or have a preference for, opiates because of their powerful action in dealing with rage, aggression and/or depression. Cocaine has its appeal because of its ability to relieve distress associated with depression, hypomania and hyperactivity. A number of clinical findings have supported the hypothesis that the preference for a specific drug is not random, but rather, appears to be a process of 'self-selection' (Dorus & Senay 1980; Rounsaville *et al.* 1982; Khantzian & Treece 1985). However, the available evidence does not support this hypothesis: no specific substances were found to alleviate specific symptoms of a particular psychiatric disorder (Dixon *et al.* 1990; Noordsy *et al.* 1991); the selection of specific psychoactive substances is not related to diagnosis (Regier *et al.* 1990); the availability factor has an influence on the selection of a specific psychoactive substance (Mueser *et al.* 1992); severely mentally ill patients use a multiple of psychoactive substances (poly-drug users) (Chen *et al.* 1992); and there is no evidence in support of the self-medication hypothesis as a necessary reinforcer of continued drug use (Castaneda *et al.* 1994).

Alleviation of dysphoria model

This model posits that severely mentally ill patients are prone to dysphoric experiences (feeling bad) that make them susceptible to the use of psychoactive substances (Birchwood *et al.* 1993). The rationale for using psychoactive substances initially is for the relief of bad feeling and to feel good (Leshner 1998) and the literature supports this notion that dysphoria motivates initial alcohol and drug use (Carey & Carey 1995; Pristach & Smith 1996; Addington & Duchak 1997). Most of the studies generally support the alleviation of dysphoria model.

Multiple risk factor model

According to Mueser *et al.* (1998), in addition to the dysphoric experiences, there are other underlying risk factors that may motivate the severe mentally ill to use psychoactive substances. The risk factors include social isolation, deficit in interpersonal skills, poor cognitive skills, educational failure, poverty, lack of adult role responsibility, association with drug subcultures and availability of illict psychoactive substances (Anthony & Helzer 1991; Berman & Noble 1993; Jones *et al.* 1994). However, there is no direct evidence for this model but the rationale for using psychoactive substances are related to the identified factors (Dixon *et al.* 1990; Noordsy *et al.* 1991).

The supersensitivity model

According to this model, 'psychobiological vulnerability, determined by a combination of genetic and environmental events, interacts with environmental stress to either precipitate the onset of a psychiatric disorder or to trigger relapse' (Mueser *et al.* 1998, p. 723). Mueser *et al.* (1998) argue that the sensitivity of psychoactive substances (increased vulnerability) may cause patients with severe mental illness to be more likely to experience negative consequences from using relatively small amounts of psychoactive substances. There are several studies that provide evidence for this model: lower levels of physical dependence (Drake *et al.* 1990; Corse *et al.* 1995); trigger of clinical symptoms by low dose of amphetamine (Lieberman *et al.* 1987); and negative clinical effects such as relapse with small quantities of alcohol or drugs (Drake *et al.* 1989). There are methodological problems associated with the research studies as many of them have focused solely on patients suffering from schizophrenia. However, according to Mueser *et al.* (1998), the supersensitivity model provides a useful theoretical framework in the understanding of how low level use of psychoactive substances often results in negative consequences in severely mentally ill patients and also the increased prevalence of drug dependence in this population.

References

Addiction Research Foundation (1986) *Essential Concepts and Strategies*. Canadian Government Publishing Centre, Supply and Services, Toronto, Canada.

Addington, J. & Duchak, V. (1997) Reasons for substance use in schizophrenia. *Acta Psychiatrica Scandinavica* **96**, 329–333.

Adityanjee, M. & Murray, R.M. (1991) The role of genetic predisposition in alcoholism. In: I.B. Glass (ed.) *The International Handbook of Addiction Behaviour*. Tavistock/Routledge, London, pp. 41–47.

Advisory Council on the Misuse of Drugs (1982) *Treatment and Rehabilitation*. HMSO, London.

Advisory Council on the Misuse of Drugs (1988) *Aids and Drug Misuse. Part 1*. HMSO, London.

Allen, K.M. (1996) Theoretical perspectives for addictions nursing practice. In: K.M. Allen (ed.) *Nursing Care of the Addicted Client*. Lippincott, Philadelphia.

American Psychiatric Association (1994) *DSM-IV: Diagnostic and Statistic Manual of Mental Disorders*, 4th edn. American Psychiatric Association, Washington DC, pp. 75–90.

Anthony, J.C. & Helzer, J.E. (1991) Syndromes of drug abuse and dependence. In: L.N. Robins & D.A. Regier (eds) *Psychiatric Disorders in America: the Epidemiologic Catchment Area Study*. Free Press, New York, pp. 116–154.

Bandura, A. (1977) *Social Learning Theory*. Prentice Hall, Englewood Cliffs, NJ.

Barnes, G. (1990) Impact of the family on adolescent drinking patterns. In: R. Collins, K. Leonard & J. Scarles (eds) *Alcohol and the Family: Research and Clinical Perspectives*. Guilford Press, New York.

Becker, H. (1966) *Outsiders: Studies in the Sociology of Deviance*. Free Press, New York.

Berman, S. & Noble, E.P. (1993) Childhood antecedents of substance misuse. *Current Opinion in Psychiatry* **6**, 382–387.

Birchwood, M., Mason, R., MacMillan, F. & Healy, J. (1993) Depression, demoralization and control over psychotic illness: A comparison of depressed and non-depressed patients with chronic psychosis. *Psychological Medicine* **23**, 387–391.

Blum, K., Noble, E.P., Sheridan, P.J. *et al.* (1990) Allelic association of human dopamine D2 receptor gene in alcoholism. *Journal of American Medical Association* **263**, 2055–2060.

Cappell, H. & Greeley (1987) Alcohol and tension reduction: An update on research and theory. In: H.T. Blane & K.E. Leonard (eds) *Psychological Theories of Drinking and Alcoholism*. Guilford Press, New York, pp. 15–22.

Carey, K.B. & Carey, M.P. (1995) Reasons for drinking among psychiatric outpatients. Relationship to drinking patterns. *Psychology of Addictive Behaviours* **9**, 251–257.

Castaneda, R., Lifshutz, H., Galanter, M. & Franco, H. (1994) Empirical assessment of the self-medication hypothesis among dually diagnosed inpatients. *Comprehensive Psychiatry* **35** (3), 180–184.

Chen, C., Balogh, M., Bathija, J., Howanitz, E., Plutchik, R. & Conte, H.R. (1992) Substance abuse among psychiatric inpatients. *Comprehensive Psychiatry* **33**, 60–64.

Christiansen, B. & Goldman, M. (1983) Alcohol related expectancies versus demographic background variables in the prediction of adolescent drinking. *Journal of Consulting and Clinical Psychology* **51**, 249–257.

Cloninger, C.R. (1987) Neurogenetic adaptive mechanisms in alcoholism. *Science* **236**, 410–415.

Collins, R. & Marlatt, G. (1981) Social modelling as a determinant of drinking behaviour: Implications for prevention and treatment. *Addictive Behaviours* **6**, 233–240.

Cook, C. (1988) The Minnesota Model in the management of drug and alcohol dependency: miracle, method or myth? Part 1. The philosophy and the programme. *British Journal of Addiction* **83**, 625–634.

Corse, S.J., Hirschinger, N.B. & Zanis, D. (1995) The use of the Addiction Severity Index with people with severe mental illness. *Psychiatric Rehabilitation Journal* **19**, 9–18.

Cummings, C., Gordon, J.R. & Marlatt, G.A. (1980) Relapse: Prevention and prediction. In: W.R. Miller (ed.) *The Addictive Behaviours: Treatment of Alcoholism, Drug Abuse, Smoking and Obesity*. Pergamon Press, New York, pp. 291–321.

Department of Health (1998) *Smoking Kills*. www.doh.gov.uk.

Dixon, L., Haas, G., Weiden, P., Sweeney, J. & Frances, A. (1990) Acute effects of drug abuse in schizophrenic patients: Clinical observations and patients' self reports. *Schizophrenia Bulletin* **16**, 69–79.

Dorus, W. & Senay, E.C. (1980) Depression, demographic dimensions and drug abuse. *American Journal of Psychiatry* **137** (6), 699–704.

Drake, R.E., Osher, F.C., Noordsy, D.L., Hurlbut, S.C., Teague, G.B. & Beaudett, M.S. (1990) Diagnosis of alcohol use disorders in schizophrenia. *Schizophrenia Bulletin* **16**, 57–67.

Drake, R.E., Osher, F.C. & Wallach, M.A. (1989) Alcohol use and abuse in schizophrenia: a prospective community study. *Journal of Nervous and Mental Disease* **177**, 408–414.

Drummond, C. (1991) Dependence on psychoactive drugs: finding a common language. In: I.B. Glass (ed.) *The International Handbook of Addiction Behaviour*. Routledge, London, Chapter 1.

Edwards, G. & Gross, M. (1976) Alcohol dependence: provisional description of a clinical syndrome. *British Journal of Addiction* **81**, 171–173.

Fields, B.P. (1999) Self-medication with alcohol and drugs by persons with severe mental illness. *Journal of the American Psychiatric Nurses Association* **5** (3), 80–87.

Fleming, N.F., Potter, D. & Kettyle, C. (1996) What are substance abuse and addiction. In: L. Friedman, N.F. Fleming, D.H. Roberts & S.E. Hyman (eds) *Source Book of Substance Abuse and Addiction*. Williams & Wilkins, Baltimore, Maryland, p. 8.

Galizio, M. & Maisto, S.A. (1985) Towards a biopsychosocial theory of substance abuse. In: M. Galizio & S.S. Maisto (eds) *Determinants of Substance Abuse: Biological, Psychological and Environmental*. Plenum Press, New York.

Ghodse, A.H. (1989) *Speciality Teaching: Psychoactive Substance Use, Disorders and Addictive Behaviour*. Submission document to St George's Hospital Medical School, London.

Ghodse, A.H. (1995) *Drugs and Addictive Behaviour*. Blackwell Science, Oxford.

Goodwin, D.W., Schulsinger, F., Knop, J., Mednick, S. & Guze, S.B. (1977) Alcoholism and depression in adopted-out daughters of alcoholics. *Archives of General Psychiatry* **34**, 751–755.

Henningfield, J.E., Cohen, C. & Slade, J.D. (1991) Is nicotine more addictive than cocaine? *British Journal of Addiction* **86** (5), 565.

Hull, J. (1981) A self-awareness model of the causes and effects of alcohol consumption. *Journal of Abnormal Psychology* **90**, 586–600.

Ikler, A. (1961) On the nature of addiction and habituation. *British Journal of Addiction* **57**, 73–79.

Institute for the Study of Drug Dependence (1996a) The Misuse of Drugs Act explained. *Revised Edition*. ISDD, London.

Institute for the Study of Drug Dependence (1996b) *Drug Abuse Briefings*, 6th edn. ISDD, London.

Jacob, T. & Leonard, K. (1988) Alcohol–spouse interaction as a function of alcoholism subtype and alcohol consumption interaction. *Journal of Abnormal Psychology* **97**, 231–237.

Jellinek, E.M. (1960) *The Disease Concept of Alcoholism*. Hillhouse Press, New Haven.

Jones, P., Guth, C., Lewis, S. & Murray, R. (1994) Low intelligence and poor education achievement precede early onset of schizophrenic psychosis. In: A.S. David & J.C. Cutting (eds) *The Neuropsychology of Schizophrenia*. Erlbaum, East Essex, UK, pp. 131–144.

Keene, J. (1997) Drug misuse. *Prevention, Harm Minimisation and Treatment*. Chapman & Hall, London, p. 180.

Khantzian, E.J. (1985) The self-medication hypothesis of addictive disorders: focus on heroin and cocaine dependence. *American Journal of Psychiatry* **142** (11), 1259–1264.

Khantzian, E.J. (1997) The self-medication hypothesis of addictive disorders: a reconsideration and recent applications. *Harvard Review of Psychiatry* **4**, 231–244.

Khantzian, E.J. & Treece, C. (1985) DSM-III psychiatric diagnosis of narcotic addicts. Recent findings. *Archives of General Psychiatry* **42** (11), 1067–1071.

Kumpter, K.L., Trunnell, E.P. & Whiteside, H.O. (1990) The biopsychosocial model: Applications to the addictions field. In: R.C. Eng (ed.) *Controversies in the Addictions Field*. Kendall/Hunt Publishing Co., Dubuque, Iowa, Vol. 1.

Leshner, A.I. (1998) Bridging the disconnect between research and practice. *The National Conference on Drug and Drug Addiction Treatment: from Research to Practice*. National Institute on Drug Abuse, Washington DC.

Lieberman, J.A., Kane, J.M. & Alvir, J. (1987) Provocative tests with psychostimulant drugs in schizophrenia. *Psychopharmacology* **91**, 415–433.

Lord President of the Council (1998) *Tackling Drugs to Build a Better Britain. The Government's Ten-Year Strategy for Tackling Drug Misuse*, Cm 3945. The Stationery Office, London.

Marks, I. (1990) Behavioural (non-chemical) addictions. *British Journal of Addiction* **85**, 1389–1394.

Marlatt, G.A., Baer, J.S., Donovan, D.M. & Kivlahan, D.R. (1988) Addictive behaviours: Etiology and treatment. *Annual Review of Psychology* **39**, 223–252.

Miller, N.S. (1991) *The Pharmacology of Alcohol and Drugs of Abuse and Addiction*. Springer-Verlag, New York.

Miller, W.R. & Hester, R.K. (1989) Treating alcohol problems: Toward an informed eclecticism. In: R.K. Hester & W.R. Miller (eds) *Handbook of Alcoholism Treatment Approaches*. Pergamon Press, New York, pp. 3–14.

Mueser, K., Bellack, A. & Blanchard, J. (1992) Comorbidity of schizophrenia and substance abuse: Implications for treatment. *Journal of Consulting and Clinical Psychology* **60** (6), 845–856.

Mueser, K.T., Drake, R.E. & Wallach, M.A. (1998) Dual diagnosis: a review of etiological theories. *Addictive Behaviours* **23** (6), 717–734.

National Institute on Alcohol Abuse and Alcoholism & Center for Substance Abuse Prevention (1993) *The Alcohol and Other Drug Thesaurus: A guide to concepts and terminology in substance abuse and addiction*. CSR Inc., Washington DC.

Noordsy, D.L., Drake, R.E., Teague, G.B. *et al.* (1991) Subjective experiences related to alcohol use among schizophrenics. *The Journal of Nervous and Mental Disease* **1179**, 410–414.

ODCCP (2000a) *World Drug Report*. Oxford University Press, Oxford.

ODCCP (2000b) Global Illicit Drug Trends 2000. www.docguide.com/crc.nst/congresses.

Orford, J. (1985) Excessive appetites. *A Psychological View of Addictions*. John Wiley & Sons, Chichester.

Pickens, R., Svikis, D., McGue, M., Lykken, D., Hesten, L. & Clayton, P. (1991) Heterogeneity in the inheritance of alcoholism. *Archives of General Psychiatry* **48** (1), 19–28.

Plant, M. (1987) *Drugs in Perspective*. Hodder and Stoughton, London, pp. 13–14.

Pristach, C.A. & Smith, C.M. (1996) Self-reported effects of alcohol use on symptoms of schizophrenia. *Psychiatric Services* **47**, 421–423.

Rassool, G. H., eds (1998) *Substance Use and Misuse: Nature, Context and Clinical Interventions*. Blackwell Science, Oxford.

Rawaf, S. & Schifano, F. (2000) The internet, children, young people and substance misuse. Editorial. *Public Health Medicine* **2** (3), 96.

Regier, D.A., Farmer, M.E., Rae, D.S., Locke, B.Z., Keith, S.J., Judd, L.L. & Goodwin, F.K. (1990) Comorbidity of mental disorders with alcohol and other drug abuse: Results from the Epidemiologic Catchment Area (ECA) study. *Journal of the American Medical Association* **264**, 2511–2518.

Rounsaville, B.J., Weissman, M.M., Wilber, C.H. & Kleber, H.D. (1982) Pathways to opiate addiction: an evaluation of differing antecedents. *British Journal of Psychiatry* **141**, 437–446.

Royal College of Psychiatrists (1987) *Drug Scenes. A report on drugs and drug dependence*. The Royal College of Psychiatrists, Gaskell, London.

Royal College of Psychiatrists and Royal College of Physicians Working Party (2000) *Drugs: Dilemmas and Choices*. Gaskell, London.

Schilit, R. & Lisansky Gomberg, E.S. (1991) *Drugs and Behaviour*. Sage Publications, Newbury Park, p. 136.

Schuckit, M.A. (1995) *Drug and Alcohol Abuse: A Clinical Guide to Diagnosis and Treatment*, 4th edn. Plenum Co., New York.

Sher, K., Walitzer, K., Wood, P. & Brent, E. (1991) Characteristics of children of alcoholics: Putative risk factors, substance use and abuse, and psychopathology. *Journal of Abnormal Psychology* **100** (4), 427–448.

Smith, J.P. (1970) Society and drugs: A short sketch. In: P.H. Blachly (ed.) *Drug Abuse Data and Debate*. Charles C. Thomas, Springfield.

Stacy, A., Widaman, K. & Marlatt, G. (1990) Expectancy models of alcohol use. *Journal of Personal and Social Psychology* **100** (4), 427–448.

Stall, R. & Biernacki, P. (1981) Addiction: some preliminary findings. *Journal of Drug Issues* **11** (3), 61–74.

Stall, R. & Biernacki, P. (1986) Spontaneous remission from the problematic use of substances: An inductive model derived from a comparative analysis of the alcohol, opiate, tobacco and food/obesity literatures. *International Journal of the Addictions* **21**, 1–32.

Statistical Bulletin (1999) Alcohol. *1976 Onwards*. Department of Health, London.

Statistical Bulletin (2000) Statistics on young people and drug misuse. *England 1998*. Department of Health, London.

Steinglass, P. (1987) *The Alcoholic Family*. Basic Books, New York.

Sullivan, E.J. (1995) *Nursing Care of Clients with Substance Abuse*. Mosby-Year Book Inc., Missouri.

Treece, C. & Khantzian, E.J. (1986) Psychodynamic factors in the development of drug dependence. *Psychiatric Clinics of North America* **9** (3), 399–412.

Tsuang, M.T., Lyons, M.J., Eisen, S.A., Goldberg, J. *et al.* (1996) Genetic influences on DSM III-R. Drug abuse and dependence. A study of 3372 pairs of twins. *American Journal of Medical Genetic* **67**, 473.

Valliant, G.E. (1983) *The Natural History of Alcoholism*. Harvard University Press, Cambridge, MA.

Wallace, J. (1977) Alcoholism from the inside out: A phenomenological analysis. In: N.J. Estes & M. Heinemann (eds) *Alcoholism: Development, Consequences and Interventions*. Mosby, St Louis.

Wallace, J. (1990) The new disease model of alcoholism. *Western Journal of Medicine* **152** (5), 502.

Wikler, A. (1948) Recent progress in research on the neurophysiological basis of morphine addiction. *American Journal of Psychiatry* **105**, 329–338.

Wikler, A. (1961) On the nature of addiction and habituation. *British Journal of Addiction* **57**, 73–79.

Wolf, P.H. (1972) Ethnic differences in alcohol sensitivity. *Science* **175**, 449–450.

World Health Organization (1969) Sixteenth report of WHO Expert Committee on Drug Dependence. Technical Report Series no. 407. WHO, Geneva.

World Health Organization (1981) Nomenclature and classification of drug- and alcohol-related problems: A WHO Memorandum. *Bulletin of the World Health Organization* **59**, 225–242.

World Health Organization (1998) *Health for all*. Data Base: European Region, WHO, Geneva.

3: Problems and Issues of Conceptualisation

Adenekan Oyefeso

Introduction

This chapter articulates the problems encountered in conceptualising the various dimensions of comorbidity of substance use and psychiatric disorders. The dimensions addressed include assessment and diagnosis, comorbidity research, and informed consent.

There are two main dimensions of comorbidity of substance use and psychiatric disorders. Comorbidity can occur where a substance use disorder (SUD) is the chronologically primary and dominant condition, underlined by at least one psychiatric disorder. The second dimension can be in the form of at least one psychiatric disorder underlined by a SUD. The challenge of determining the chronologically primary disorder remains a major challenge for clinicians, especially where both disorders have independent courses. Also, it is increasingly becoming a norm for substance misuse and mental health professionals to define dominance of a disorder in terms of the first treatment episode or agency of first presentation, substance misuse service or mental health team.

Irrespective of chronology and dominance, patients with concurrent psychiatric disorder and SUD are known to experience higher levels of psychiatric, medical and social complications. These include high rates of relapse and re-hospitalisation (Linszen *et al.* 1994), tendency to suicide (Bartels *et al.* 1992); violence (Cuffel *et al.* 1994); arrests and incarceration (Abram & Teplin 1991); homelessness (Drake *et al.* 1991); and family problems (Dixon *et al.* 1995).

Compared to singly diagnosed psychiatric patients, dual disorder patients are generally less stable, experiencing more severe symptomatology, higher hospitalisation rates (Maynard & Cox 1998); higher frequency of arrests (Clark *et al.* 1999); and poorer housing stability (Osher *et al.* 1994). The heightened instability in psychiatric, medical and social status of these patients emphasises the need for thorough understanding of the concept of comorbidity.

Diagnosis

One of the main challenges facing clinicians involved in the care of patients with comorbid disorders is inaccuracy of diagnosis. Diagnosis serves two main functions—definition of clinical entities and determination of treatment (Spitzer 1976). This chapter focuses on the former.

The concept of definition of clinical entities is based on the premise that patients with the same diagnosis don't always describe identical features, but must always present with a number of common cardinal symptoms. Such presentations should describe a similar natural history—similar age of onset, life course, prognosis and complications (Maxmen & Ward 1995). For example, the emergence of alcohol dependence and schizophrenia in an 18-year-old man can be a result of different aetiological factors.

Both disorders can be genetically transmitted. They can be precipitated by common psychosocial factors and can be aggravated by biological, psychological or environmental conditions.

Diagnostic manuals

Appropriate use of diagnostic manuals such as the DSM-IV (American Psychiatric Association 1994), which presents multiaxial diagnosis, can facilitate understanding of the concept of comorbidity. There are five axes in all, described as follows:

Axis I: Clinical syndromes, developmental disorders and other conditions of clinical relevance.

Axis II: This includes personality disorders and traits, and learning difficulties.

Axis III: This relates to general medical conditions and physical symptoms associated with the current psychiatric problem.

Axis IV: Describes psychosocial and environmental problems.

Axis V: This is the Global Assessment of Functioning (GAF).

Axes I and II disorders are the focus of this chapter, given that the majority of SUD and psychiatric disorder comorbidities belong to these categories. The main forms of co-occurrence are discussed below.

Axis I comorbidity

SUD and schizophrenia

There is increasing evidence that lifetime prevalence rates of SUD among schizophrenic patients range between 40% and 70% (Mueser *et al.* 1995; Dixon 1999), with an earlier onset of psychotic symptoms in substance abusing schizophrenics (George & Krystal 2000). Patients in this category are more likely to be young males (Mueser *et al.* 1999).

SUD and mood disorders

Similarly, prevalence rates of SUD among patients with mood disorders range between 50% and 70% (Mueser *et al.* 1999). Between 30 and 50% of opioids abusing/dependent patients are known to meet the criteria for lifetime major depressive disorder (Kaplan *et al.* 1994, p. 391). Furthermore, opiate addicts record a higher rate of suicide than the general population (Oyefeso *et al.* 1999). However, SUD is less common in unipolar than in bipolar disorders (Lynskey 1998). Among cocaine abusers, lifetime and current prevalence rates of mood disorder are about 61% and 445, respectively, while lifetime prevalence of major depression in this group is about 31% (Rounsaville *et al.* 1991).

SUD and anxiety disorders

The rates of anxiety disorders among alcoholic patients range between 10% and 69% (Kushner *et al.* 1990); social phobia being the most commonly observed condition in this patient population.

Arriving at a diagnosis of Axis I comorbidity can be challenging.

First, drug intoxication can often mimic acute psychotic episodes. Acute cannabis intoxication may result in anxiety states that manifest as panic attacks and fears of unspecified origins.

Second, drug-induced psychotic disorders can be misdiagnosed as acute episodes of severe mental illness. For instance, cocaine-induced psychotic disorder, often characterised by paranoid delusions, auditory hallucinations, and, less often, by inappropriate sexual behaviour, and violence can be mistaken for an acute phase of paranoid schizophrenia.

Third, signs and symptoms of intoxication on, and withdrawal from, a substance are sometimes identical to symptoms of a psychiatric disorder. Cocaine-induced mood disorder is a good example of this problem. Cocaine intoxication is identical to a hypomanic state, while symptoms of cocaine withdrawal such as lethargy; tearfulness; suicidal ideation, etc. are similar to those of major depression.

Axis I and II comorbidity

This type of comorbidity describes the co-occurrence of SUD and personality disorders (PDs). The prevalence rates of DSM-III-R DSM-IV Axis II PDs among patients with SUD range between 30% and 90% (Oyefeso *et al.* 1998; Verheul & van den Brink 2000). The PDs mostly affected are paranoid (Cluster A); antisocial, borderline (Cluster B); and avoidant (Cluster C) types. Given the nature of problematic substance use and dependence, and the chaotic lifestyle of drug addicts in general, there is a strong overlap between the symptomatology of some personality disorders and behavioural patterns of drug addicts. DSM-IV criteria for antisocial personality disorder (APD) and borderline personality disorder (BPD) illustrate this point.

SUD and APD

Drug addicts largely fulfil all six category-A criteria for DSM-IV APD:

(1) Failure to conform to social norms.

(2) Impulsivity or failure to plan ahead.

(3) Irritability and aggressiveness, as indicated by repeated physical assaults.

(4) Reckless disregard for safety of self and colleagues.

(5) Consistent irresponsibility, as indicated by repeated failure to sustain consistent work behaviour or honour financial obligations.

(6) Lack of remorse, as indicated by being indifferent to, or rationalising, having hurt, mistreated, or stolen from another.

It is therefore, not uncommon, after history-taking, for clinicians to assume that a patient with APD is a drug-abusing patient. The crucial criterion most likely to be overlooked by clinicians is evidence of conduct disorder with onset before the age of 15 years. Generally, many cases of conduct problems in childhood, though acknowledged, never receive a formal diagnosis of conduct disorder. Consequently, the prevalence of APD among patients with SUD can be an overestimate. Appropriate application of the principles of differential diagnosis would indicate that many problematic substance users frequently engage in antisocial behaviours, and therefore, would readily fulfil the criteria for adult antisocial behaviour rather than APD.

SUD and BPD

Many symptoms of BPD overlap with the behavioural characteristics of problematic substance users. The most frequently encountered symptoms clinically are as follows:

• A pattern of unstable and intense interpersonal relationships characterised by alternating between extremes of idealisation and devaluation. (This cyclical pattern may be precipitated by intoxication and withdrawal from stimulant drugs.)

• Impulsivity. (This symptom also includes substance abuse.)

• Recurrent suicidal behaviour, gestures or threats. (These can occur frequently during withdrawal from cocaine or as part of an underlying mood disorder that characterises many addicts.)

• Affective instability. (This may or may not be drug-induced.)

• Inappropriate, intense anger or difficulty controlling anger. (This may be due to substance intoxication.)

Implications of interaction between concurrent disorders

The overlap in symptomatology between SUD and other disorders calls for careful assessment and diagnostic efficiency. First, the clinician needs to be aware of the complex interplay between Axis I disorders in general, which are more florid presentations, and Axis II, which are more chronic in form. Consistent recourse to differential diagnosis can prove useful in preventing misdiagnosis.

In order to improve the conceptualisation of comorbidity, there is a need to explore the accuracy of diagnoses made and specify the chronology of the diagnosed disorders. Three criteria for facilitating this effort are:

(1) diagnostic stability;

(2) developmental course; and

(3) family history (Alterman & Cacciola 1991).

Diagnostic stability

Diagnostic interviews must take into account the stability of presenting symptoms, and the accuracy of information provided by the patient. Age of onset and duration of symptoms are essential elements for distinguishing between chronologically primary and secondary disorders. Acute symptoms of drug-induced disorders often colour symptoms of comorbid Axis I disorders. In this instance, assessment should involve close observation to allow for remission of florid symptoms.

Thereafter, the age of onset, periods of remission and symptom offset, and duration of enduring symptoms should offer meaningful diagnostic information. In the case of personality disorders, the clinician should be cognisant of the patient's functioning over the entire lifetime, and avoid the distraction of the drug abusing patient's level of functioning in the period prior to assessment, often characterised by a mesh of florid symptoms. From the above, it is obvious that chronology of diagnoses cannot be established during initial assessment. Continuous, or ongoing comprehensive assessment therefore should be the norm.

Furthermore, at initial assessment, problematic substance users may present inaccurate histories as a result of intoxication or impaired memory, or may deliberately falsify information. Ongoing comprehensive assessment therefore requires collateral detailed information from the referring agencies and significant others.

Developmental course

Establishing the chronology of comorbid disorders is essential for making accurate diagnosis, and devising an appropriate treatment plan. Specification of the age of onset and determination of sequelae of the disorders are essential. Details of present illness, past psychiatric illness, and development history should enable the construction of onset of each of the co-occurring disorders, and also of the aetiology of these conditions. Quite often, the presenting condition can be a sequela of an underlying psychopathology. Acute psychiatric symptoms can be direct effects of drugs (e.g. hypomania due to cocaine intoxication); substance withdrawal (e.g. alcohol hallucinosis); or of independent medical problems or physical complications of substance misuse (e.g. HIV/AIDS and its pathophysiological implications). Assessment therefore should involve medical, neurological and toxicological investigations so that the complex interaction between the chronologically primary disorder and its sequelae can be better understood.

Family history

Information on the family history of psychiatric illness is particularly important in discerning the overlap between SUD and personality disorders, given the enduring level of functioning required for diagnosing the latter. From both cross-sectional and time line consideration of the emergence of symptoms, and given the relatively enduring nature of personality disorders, one can always assume that personality disorders precede SUD. However, this is not always the case, especially with patients who are family history positive (FHP) for SUD, notably alcoholism.

The mechanism of the influence of family history on chronology of comorbid disorders is still unclear. Alterman and Cacciola (1991) have presented a summary of research that demonstrates the complex link between FHP alcoholism and antisocial personality disorder (APD):

• There is a likelihood of family history of APD and addiction among APD addicts (intergenerational concurrence).

• Alcoholic patients with a higher density of FHP alcoholism are also more likely to meet the criteria for APD diagnosis (alcoholism as chronological primary disorder).

• The presence of APD in the family may heighten the risk of alcoholism among family members (APD as chronological primary disorder).

Investigating comorbidity

Studies of comorbidity are often conducted in three types of setting: *high risk populations, general practice* and the *general population*. Studies of high risk populations include clinical populations of substance misusers and/or severely mentally ill patients, the homeless, etc. Irrespective of the population investigated, the focus of study needs to be specified, e.g. determining the prevalence and pattern of borderline personality disorder and symptomatology among opiate addicts. The findings of such studies are only generalisable to such specific populations. Sources of data for this type of studies include hospital admission charts, local case registers and face-to-face case identification interviews.

General practice records are also a useful source of data. They provide data on presenting symptomatology, diagnostic impressions, and prescribing patterns of psychotropic medication.

General population surveys examine the distribution of comorbid disorders in the entire population, and the detection of cases that have not presented to treatment services. Examples of such surveys are the Epidemiologic Catchment Area (ECA) study (Robins & Regier 1991), the National Comorbidity Survey (Kessler *et al*. 1994) and the National Psychiatric Morbidity surveys of Great Britain (Meltzer *et al*. 1995).

Problems of comorbidity studies

Some of the problems with comorbidity studies are inherent in the data sources. Hospital charts are useful only for obtaining prevalence estimates on cases presenting for treatment in the National Health Service (NHS); they usually exclude patients treated in the private sector. Furthermore, the accuracy of the prevalence estimates depends largely on clinicians' ability to currently identify and classify cases, and to make accurate records in the charts.

The problem with case registers centres around the absence of standard procedures for collecting diagnostic information in psychiatric services (Jenkins *et al*. 1997), and across substance misuse services. Data from face-to-face interviews rely on the patient's ability to recall relevant diagnostic information accurately, a circumstance that is further determined by the presence or absence of substance effects, intoxication and/or withdrawal. The validity of general practice consultation data is strongly influenced, among other things, by the wide diagnostic variation across practices, and by the extent of utilisation of primary care services.

Carefully planned general population or community surveys are usually representative of the general population. The problem with them, however, lies in the variation in the sensitivity, specificity, and validity of the survey instruments used within and across populations, which in turn affect the accuracy of the estimates reported.

Another source of inaccuracy is the variation in the ability and experience of interviewers in both substance misuse and mental health, and in the sequence and range of disorders investigated. Poor interviewing skills and biased questioning always yield spurious estimates, even if there is consistency in interview personnel.

Finally, there are inherent limitations in the validity of the range and severity of disorders identified in general population surveys. Regier *et al*. (1988) have suggested that high prevalence rates in such surveys can be attributed to transient 'homeostatic responses to internal or external stimuli (such as blood pressure, interview anxiety, etc.) that do not represent the psychopathologic disorders' (p. 5).

Bearing these problems in mind, clinicians must ensure that they scrutinise the findings of comorbidity studies vigorously, to ensure that accurate information is being used to enhance practice.

Informed consent

Consent has been defined as:
    'the voluntary and continuing permission of the patient to receive a
    particular treatment, based on adequate knowledge of the purpose,

nature, likely effects and risks of that treatment, including the likelihood of its success and any alternatives to it.'(Department of Health 1993, 15.12)

Although the concept of informed consent, and its application in clinical practice, is well established in SUD and psychiatric disorders, there may be a need to explore the way this concept applies to comorbid disorders.

Given the difficulty in determining the distinctiveness of overlapping disorders, it seems that there is insufficient evidence on treatment effectiveness. Consequently, it may seem that the tenets of informed consent are being violated.

Hatcher (1995) has argued that the reason many patients consent to pharmacotherapy is to reduce the risk of recurrence of the acute phase of their illness, rather than as a result of careful independent consideration, by the patient, of the effectiveness and side-effects of prescribed medication.

Second, there is evidence that many psychiatric patients suffer from cognitive abnormalities (Goldberg *et al.* 1993; Jones 1995) that may put their capability to grant consent in doubt. Given the toxic confusional states induced by substances with abuse liability, such cognitive impairments can be more profound in patients with comorbid disorders. Consequently, there is a need to review existing protocols on informed consent, and to provide additional support to patients to assist in making informed decisions about treatment.

Conclusion

The problems and issues relating to recognition, diagnosis and assessment, differential diagnosis and natural history of comorbid substance use and psychiatric disorders have been explored. It is becoming increasingly important that patients with dual problems provide a great challenge to practitioners in the field. In this era of evidence-based practice, it is essential for practitioners to enhance their skills for evaluating research, ensuring that the 'evidence' that they adopt for practice has been scrutinised for reliability and validity. Furthermore, with the introduction of the Human Rights Act in the United Kingdom, it has become necessary for practitioners to revisit the tenets of informed consent and ensure that its principles are strictly adhered to.

References

Abram, K.M. & Teplin, L.A. (1991) Co-occurring disorders among mentally ill jail detainees: Implications for public policy. *American Psychologist* **46**, 1036–1045.

Alterman, A.I. & Cacciola, J.S. (1991) The antisocial personality disorder diagnosis in substance abusers. *Problems and Issues. Journal of Nervous and Mental Disorders* **179**, 401–409.

American Psychiatric Association (1994) *Diagnostic and Statistical Manual*, 4th edn. American Psychiatric Press, Washington DC.

Bartels, S.J., Drake, R.E. & McHugo, G.J. (1992) Alcohol abuse, depression, and suicidal behaviour in schizophrenia. *American Journal of Psychiatry* **149**, 394–395.

Clark, R.E., Ricketts, S.K. & McHugo, G.J. (1999) Legal system involvement and costs for persons in treatment for severe mental illness and substance use disorders. *Psychiatric Services* **50**, 641–647.

Cuffel, B.J., Shumway, M., Chouljian, T.L. & MacDonald, T. (1994) A longitudinal study of substance use and community violence in schizophrenia. *Journal of Nervous and Mental Disease* **182**, 704–708.

Department of Health (1993) Code of Practice of the Mental Health Act 1983. London.

Dixon, J.M. (1999) Psychological interventions for schizophrenia. *Effective Health Care* **6**, 3.

Dixon, L., McNary, S. & Lehman, A. (1995) Substance abuse and family relationships of persons with severe mental illnesses. *American Journal of Psychiatry* **152**, 456–458.

Drake, R.E., Mercer-McFadden, C., Mueser, K.T., McHugo, G.J. & Bond, G.R. (1998) Review of integrated mental health and substance abuse treatment for patients with dual disorders. *Schizophrenic Bulletin* **24**, 589–608.

Drake, R.E., Osher, F.C. & Wallach, M.A. (1991) Homelessness and dual diagnosis. *American Psychologist* **46**, 1149–1158.

George, T.P. & Krystal, J.H. (2000) Comorbidity of psychiatric and substance abuse disorders. *Current Opinion in Psychiatry* **13**(3), 327–331.

Goldberg, T.E., Torrey, E.F., Gold, T.M. *et al.* (1993) Learning and memory in monozygotic twins discordant for schizophrenia. *Psychological Medicine* **23**, 71–85.

Hatcher, S. (1995) Decision analysis in psychiatry. *British Journal of Psychiatry* **166**, 184–190.

Jenkins, R., Bebbington, P., Brugha, T. *et al.* (1997) The national psychiatric morbidity surveys of Great Britain — Strategy and methods. *Psychological Medicine* **27**, 765–774.

Jones, G.H. (1995) Consent in chronic schizophrenia? *British Journal of Psychiatry* **167**, 565–568.

Kaplan, H.I., Sadock, B.J. & Grebb, J.A. (1994) *Synopsis of Psychiatry.* Williams & Wilkins, Philadelphia, pp. 383–456.

Kessler, R.C., McGonagle, K.A., Zhao, S. *et al.* (1994) Lifetime and 12-month prevalence of DSM-III-R psychiatric disorders in the United States. *Archives of General Psychiatry* **51**, 8–19.

Kushner, M.G., Sher, K.J. & Beitman, B.D. (1990) The reaction between alcohol problems and the anxiety disorders. *American Journal of Psychiatry* **147**, 687.

Linszen, D.H., Dingemans, P.M. & Lenior, M.E. (1994) Cannabis abuse and the course of recent-onset schizophrenia. *Archives of General Psychiatry* **51**, 273–279.

Lynskey, M.T. (1998) The comorbidity of alcohol dependence and affective disorders: treatment implications. *Drug and Alcohol Dependence* **52**, 201–209.

Maxmen, J.S. & Ward, N.G. (1995) *Essential Psychopathology and its Treatment*, 2nd edn. WW Norton, New York, p. 4.

Maynard, C. & Cox, G.B. (1998) Psychiatric hospitalization of persons with dual diagnosis: Estimates from two national surveys. *Psychiatric Services* **49**, 1615–1617.

Meltzer, H., Gill, B., Pettigrew, M. & Hinds, K. (1995) *OPCS Surveys of Psychiatric Morbidity Report 1. The Prevalence of Psychiatric Morbidity Among Adults Aged 16–64 Living in Private Households in Great Britain.* HMSO, London.

Mueser, K.T., Bennett, M. & Kushner, M.G. (1995) Epidemiology of substance use disorders among persons with chronic mental illnesses. In: A.F. Lehman & L. Dixon (eds) *Double Jeopardy: Chronic Mental Illness and Substance Abuse.* Harwood Academic Publishers, New York, pp. 9–25.

Mueser, K.T., Rosenberg, S.D., Drake, R.E. *et al.* (1999) Conduct disorder, antisocial personality disorder and substance abuse disorders in schizophrenia and major affective disorders. *Journal of Studies on Alcohol* **60**, 278–284.

Osher, F.C., Drake, R.E., Noordsy, D.L. *et al.* (1994) Correlates and outcomes of alcohol use disorder among rural schizophrenic outpatients. *Journal of Clinical Psychiatry* **55**, 109–113.

Oyefeso, A., Ghodse, H., Clancy, C. & Corkery, J. (1999) Suicide among drug addicts in the United Kingdom. *British Journal of Psychiatry* **175**, 277–282.

Oyefeso, A., Ghodse, H., Crawford, Clancy, C. & Byrne, S. (1998) Comorbidity of personality disorders in opiate addicts. *Chinese Journal of Drug Dependence* **7**, 110–114.

Regier, D.A., Hirschfeld, R.M., Goodwin, F.K. *et al.* (1988) The NIMH depression awareness, recognition, and treatment program: structure, aims, and scientific basis. *American Journal of Psychiatry* **145**, 1351–1357.

Robins, L.N. & Regier, D.A., eds (1991) Psychiatric disorders in America. *The Epidemiological Catchment Area Study*. The Free Press, New York.

Rounsaville, B.J., Anton, S.F., Carroll, K., Budde, D., Prusoff, B.A. & Gawin, F. (1991) Psychiatric diagnoses of treatment-seeking cocaine abusers. *Archives of General Psychiatry* **48**, 45.

Spitzer, R.L. (1976) More on pseudoscience in science and the case for psychiatric diagnosis: a critique of Rosenhan's 'On being sane in insane places' and 'The contextual nature of psychiatric diagnosis'. *Archives of General Psychiatry* **137**, 151–164.

Verheul, R. & van den Brink, W. (2000) The role of personality pathology in the aetiology and treatment of substance use disorders. *Current Opinion in Psychiatry* **13**, 163–169.

4: Psychiatric Disorders and Substance Misuse: Psychopathology

C.A. Harrison and M.T. Abou Saleh

Introduction

Since the early 1990s it has become increasingly recognised that there is a common co-occurrence of psychiatric disorders with alcohol and drug use disorders, which has a profound impact on theoretical and conceptual issues in the study of psychopathology and poses significant problems regarding assessment and treatment. The aetiology of this high prevalence is unclear and opinions have varied on the reasons for this comorbidity, an association most commonly explained by either a causal relationship or shared aetiological factor underlying both disorders. Attention has been focused on this common phenomenon, leading to improved diagnostic instruments and further research on the complex relationships between a wide variety of psychiatric conditions and substance misuse. The present chapter describes the prevalence and natural history of the co-occurrence of substance and psychiatric disorders, modes of transmission, overview of diagnostic methods and psychopathology of specific disorders commonly encountered in clinical practice.

Epidemiological studies on comorbidity of substance use and psychiatric disorders

Community based populations

There are three major community based studies: the Epidemiological Catchment Area Study (ECA)(Regier *et al.* 1984), the National Comorbidity Survey (NCS)(Kessler *et al.* 1994) and the National Longitudinal Alcohol Epidemiological Survey (NLAES)(Grant 1995).

The ECA estimates of the prevalence of lifetime disorders were 22.5% for all mental disorders other than alcohol or drug use disorders and 16% for substance use disorders (Regier *et al.* 1984). The most common disorders were anxiety disorders (14.6%) and affective disorders (8.3%). A respondent with any lifetime mental disorder, had a significantly greater chance of also experiencing an alcohol or drug use disorder, with an odds ratio (OR) (a measure indicating the strength of association between disorders where a ratio greater than 1 is statistically significant) for any mental disorder and drug use disorder of 4.5 and for any mental disorder and alcohol use disorder of 2.3.

Information was also available on lifetime and current (preceding 6 months) comorbidity for specific mental disorders. The OR indicating the association of schizophrenia with any substance use disorder was 4.0, broken down further into an odds ratio of 3.8 for alcohol and 6.2 for drug disorder. The ORs for anxiety disorders and substance use disorders were lower, with the exception of panic disorder. Bipolar 1 disorder had a higher level of association than other affective disorders, with an OR of 7.9 for any substance use, and an OR of 2.6 for any lifetime affective disorder. The presence of a drug use disorder greatly increased the odds of having an alcohol use disorder with an odds ratio of 7.1.

The NCS (Kessler *et al.* 1994) showed overall higher prevalence rates for many disorders than that found in the ECA, with the lifetime prevalence of any mental disorder, including substance disorders being as high as 48%. The OR indicating the association between nonaffective psychosis and alcohol disorders was 2.2 and between nonaffective psychosis and drug disorders, 2.7. The OR for anxiety disorders and substance disorders ranged from 2.2 (phobia)–3.2 (post traumatic stress disorder, PTSD). The OR for Bipolar 1 and substance use disorders was 4.9 for both alcohol and drug use disorders. These are all lower rates than those found in the ECA, but when current (preceding 6 months) prevalence was examined, comorbidity was higher than found in the ECA. The association of current drug and alcohol use disorders was very high (OR=20.6)

The National Longitudinal Alcohol Epidemiological Study was conducted in 1992 (Grant 1995), and focused on alcohol, drug and depressive disorder. The results showed a high level of association between alcohol and drug use disorders, confirming that seen in previous studies such as the NCA. The current prevalence of depression found in this sample was 3.3%, whilst the lifetime prevalence was 9.9%. Odds ratios showed a significant association between drug use and depression (7.2, current, 5.2, lifetime) and alcohol abuse and depression (3.7, current, 3.6, lifetime).

Clinical populations

Studies of the prevalence of psychiatric disorders in clinical populations in drug and alcohol treatment settings, have reported remarkably high rates of comorbidity (Penick *et al.* 1988; Rounsaville *et al.* 1991). There is considerable controversy about the methods used for diagnosis of comorbid psychiatric disorders in patients with substance misuse. Issues include the presence and meaning of primary and secondary disorders when defined by age at first onset, the reliability of diagnosis of comorbidity and whether comorbid disorders are independent, substance induced or syndromes that mimic psychiatric symptoms but are actually the expected effects of alcohol or drug intoxication or withdrawal.

Psychiatric diagnostic studies in samples of treatment seeking substance abusers have produced widely varying estimates of prevalence, especially for mood and anxiety disorders. It is likely that this is largely due to inconsistencies in the methods and criteria used to differentiate psychiatric disorders from the effects, both acute and chronic of substance use. The terms primary and secondary have been used to describe comorbid psychiatric syndromes in substance misusers, usually to imply cause and effect between the substance use and co-occurring disorder. However, the pathophysiology of mental disorders is not sufficiently understood to make this judgement, as there are no empirical methods available to determine primary or secondary in the causal sense. Psychiatric disorders tend to have characteristic ages of onset, with conduct disorders and attention deficit disorders (ADD) beginning in childhood, alcohol and other substance abuse beginning in early to mid adolescence, and mood and anxiety disorders beginning in adolescence and adulthood.

Feigner defines primary–secondary as indicating the age of onset of the disorder (Feigner *et al*. 1972), the disorder with earliest age of onset being called primary. This can probably be measured reliably through standard structured interviews but may not be helpful in distinguishing whether the secondary disorder is independent of the first or how the two are related. Thus conduct/antisocial personality disorders and ADD can usually be chronologically primary and mood and anxiety disorders chronologically secondary due to their age of onset. There have been studies, which demonstrate concurrent and predictive validity of the chronological distinction. Schuckit (1983) showed that alcoholics with secondary depression tend to resemble non-depressed alcoholics more than they resemble primary depressives, and that their depressive symptoms remit after detoxification from alcohol whereas depressive symptoms in primary depressives persist despite detoxification (Brown *et al*. 1995). However, interestingly both primary (McGrath *et al*. 1996) and secondary (Mason *et al*. 1996) depression in alcoholics appear to respond to antidepressant medication, thus the chronological primary–secondary distinction may have limited validity in predicting treatment response.

Diagnostic instruments

There have been important developments in the production of structured diagnostic instruments, with greater reliability and validity for the diagnosis of comorbid mental illness and substance use disorder. The Psychiatric Research Interview for Substance and Mental Disorders (PRISM) was designed to overcome reliability problems in the diagnosis of comorbid psychiatric disorders in substance user populations (Hasin *et al*. 1996). The substance use disorder sections are at the beginning of the interview allowing a thorough knowledge of the subject's pattern and history of substance use before asking questions about the presence of mood and other mental disorders. Reliability studies have shown high kappa values (agreement greater than chance), which have been substantially better than those found with studies using other diagnostic interviews in substance user populations.

DSM-IV places more emphasis on comorbidity than previous versions, producing three categories:

(1) primary;

(2) substance-induced; and

(3) expected effects of substances.

It also provides guidelines for distinguishing comorbid syndromes in the setting of ongoing substance use. For instance, primary major depression is diagnosed if one of the following three criteria is met:

(1) Persistence of mood symptoms for more than four weeks after the end of substance intoxication or acute substance withdrawal.

(2) The development of mood symptoms that are substantially in excess to what would be expected given the type or amount of substance used or the duration of use, or

(3) a history of prior recurrent primary episodes of Major Depression (American Psychiatric Association 1994).

'Substance-induced' disorders are diagnosed when symptoms of the disorder are present, having developed during or within a month of substance intoxication or withdrawal, the requirements for 'primary major depression', stated above are not met but the symptoms are in 'excess' of those usually associated with the intoxication or withdrawal syndrome and are severe enough to warrant independent clinical attention.

If neither primary or substance-induced criteria are met, the syndrome is diagnosed as *substance intoxication* or *withdrawal* (American Psychiatric Association 1994). In conclusion, DSM-IV expands on the notion of primary disorders to include persistence during abstinence and the occurrence of a syndrome during substance use that could not be merely attributed to the effects of the substance in question. This advance allows the recognition that mood or other psychiatric syndromes developing during substance use may have clinical implications despite being chronologically secondary, either by influencing outcome of addiction treatment or by being responsive to psychotropic medication.

Improved diagnostic instruments have allowed more valid studies in both community and clinical populations confirming high levels of comorbidity of psychiatric disorders and substance use disorders. A number of studies showed high rates of comorbidity between alcoholism and anxiety disorders (Woodruff *et al.* 1972; Ross *et al.* 1988), affective disorders (Merikangas & Gerlernter 1990) and antisocial personality disorder (Powell *et al.* 1982). Similarly substance misuse in general was shown to be strongly comorbid with major depression, bipolar, antisocial personality disorder and anxiety disorders (Chitwood 1985; Rounsaville *et al.* 1991) in clinically treated samples of opiate and cocaine users.

Aetiology of comorbidity

A number of aetiological models for comorbidity have been introduced: *common factor* models, *secondary misuse* models and *psychiatric illness* models. The categories of substance misuse and psychiatric disorder comorbidity are shown in Table 4.1.

The common factor models include the model for common genetic factors and antisocial personality disorder. Studies have not supported the common genetic factor in the causation of substance misuse and psychiatric disorder. However the presence of antisocial personality disorder was shown to be a common factor in its causation. Patients with severe mental illness and antisocial personality disorder are more likely to have substance misuse than patients with no antisocial personality disorder. Morever patients who also had conduct disorder in childhood as well as antisocial personality disorder in adulthood were at higher risk for comorbidity. Mueser *et al.* (2000) in a cohort study involving 325 patients with comorbid psychiatric disorder and substance misuse identified predictors of comorbidity: male gender, young age, less education, criminal activity, conduct and antisocial personality disorder.

Secondary substance misuse models include the models of self-medication, alleviation of dysphoria and supersensitivity.

The self-medication model depicts that psychiatric patients use specific substance to alleviate specific symptoms. This notion has not been supported by evidence with non-specific improvement with the use of alcohol or drugs. On the contrary, psychiatric patients who use alcohol and drugs have worse outcomes. The alleviation of dysphoria model however, has more credence although dysphoria is associated with a general proneness to addiction rather than the use of any specific substance.

The supersensitivity model is supported by the observation that patients with severe mental illness show high sensitivity to low doses of alcohol and drugs, particularly amphetamine, which precipitate a relapse in their illness.

The secondary psychiatric illness model draws upon the kindling/behavioural sensitisation hypothesis, e.g. drug use may precipitate schizophrenia or other psychotic disorders with an earlier age of onset than is the case with those who have not used drugs. Substance misuse has been shown to be as-

Table 4.1 Categories of substance misuse and psychiatric disorder comorbidity

Primary substance misuse with secondary psychiatric disorder, e.g.
  alcohol dependence with secondary depression, amphetamine induced psychosis
Primary psychiatric disorder with secondary substance misuse, e.g.
  self-medication with drugs/alcohol
Concurrent/dual primary substance misuse and psychiatric disorder, e.g.
  cocaine misuse and bipolar affective disorder
Common aetiological factor causing substance misuse and psychiatric disorder, e.g.
  antisocial personality disorder (APD) with cannabis misuse and schizophrenia

sociated with poor outcome in bipolar affective disorder and poor response to lithium prophylaxis. Moreover specific drugs may cause specific psychiatric disorders, e.g. amphetamine or cocaine induced psychosis with distinct features of predominant paranoid and affective symptoms and fewer negative symptoms of schizophrenia. The one neuro-imaging study reported fewer standard MRI abnormalities in schizophrenic patients with substance misuse than patients with schizophrenia only.

Psychiatric disorders secondary to substance use

Psychopathology can occur as the expected effects of substance use and can vary depending on the substance used. Psychiatric symptoms from alcohol and drug disorders occur more commonly than comorbid psychiatric disorders in addicted patients, but can be difficult to distinguish. The following paragraphs examine the psychopathology that can be produced independently of comorbid psychiatric diagnosis by the use of stimulants, cannabis, and alcohol.

Stimulants: cocaine and amphetamines

Up to 80% of regular cocaine users experience symptoms, which are indistinguishable from hypomania, with symptoms such as euphoria, grandiosity, impulsiveness, impaired judgement and marked psychomotor activity, usually subsiding within half an hour. The user may experience hallucinations, both visual and auditory similar to those seen in schizophrenia, along with the more classical tactile hallucinations such as formication (the feelings of insects under the skin). Aggressive behaviour and panic may result from paranoid feelings. Prolonged or high dose use may lead to a toxic psychosis with persecutory delusions and hallucinations and a loss of insight, a condition which usually subsides within 24 h but may be indistinguishable from acute psychosis of other causes.

Amphetamines may produce similar toxic reactions, the psychosis may last longer than that produced by cocaine, but will usually resolve within a few days (Connell 1958). This condition usually occurs in long-term users, but may occur after a single use. It starts a day or two after use and consists of disordered thinking, hallucinations and paranoid ideas, and the production of random, pointless, repetitive behaviour such as involuntary picking and scratching at the skin.

Cocaine stimulates the brain by altering the balance of the chemical messenger dopamine. Amphetamine has a similar structure to noradrenaline and dopamine, producing similar pharmacological effects to that of cocaine, but with a longer duration of action. Both stimulate a particular bundle of dopamine containing nerves, which are central to the drug's ability to produce a 'high', but can ultimately produce depletion of dopamine stores in this reward system. This imbalance of dopamine is similar to that found in patients with schizophrenia, and may be involved in the production of the psychopathology seen in drug-induced psychosis.

In the United States, acute psychological and physical illnesses resulting from cocaine use account for 20% of all admissions to emergency treatment rooms (Cregler & Mark 1986). In the mid 1980s 20% of people who committed suicide in New York were found to have cocaine in their bodies and an analysis of 300 psychiatric inpatients showed that 64% could be diagnosed as substance misusers, with more than half misusing cocaine. This trend is starting to be more evident in the United Kingdom, especially in inner city acute psychiatric services.

Cannabis

The consumption of cannabis can lead to the development of a wide range of psychopathology, including the production commonly of anxiety and panic attacks. Symptoms are usually brief in duration and may include restlessness, depersonalisation, derealisation, paranoia and transient mood disorders (Thomas 1993). High doses or prolonged consumption may produce an acute toxic confusional state, which is usually transient and self-limiting. There is substantial variation in the prevalence figures for acute psychotic reactions to cannabis, which may be explained by variation in the strength and type of cannabis consumed. Some acute psychotic reactions occur in clear consciousness and are indistinguishable from schizophrenia-like psychosis. It is difficult to differentiate whether these illnesses are in fact relapses in previously psychotic patients who use cannabis, precipitated in patients who are vulnerable or actual reactions produced by ingestion of cannabis. There is no conclusive evidence that cannabis can cause long-term psychiatric illness, or is an independent risk factor for schizophrenia.

Cannabis can also produce affective disturbances, which are usually mild and transient episodes of low mood. There has been no evidence that it can precipitate more serious or prolonged mood disorders. The term 'amotivational syndrome' was devised in the 1990s to describe a cluster of symptoms thought to occur in regular cannabis users, which include apathy, loss of ambition and determination, impaired concentration and deterioration in academic performance which can present as an apparent personality change. However, studies have been inconclusive and the probable explanation is that of chronic intoxication rather than deterioration of personality.

Alcohol

Alcohol can produce a wide range of psychopathology as a result of intoxication, withdrawal and dependence with both acute and chronic effects. Glass and Jackson (1988) found that 10% of psychiatric patients have an alcohol problem, and 40% of these patients also had a diagnosis of additional psychiatric diagnosis. Alcohol abuse can often lead to the symptoms of depression, such as low mood, agitation, apathy, suicidal ideation, loss of libido, early morning waking, loss of appetite and weight loss. The relationship between alcohol and suicide is well established, and 15% of alcoholic patients may eventually commit suicide (Hawton 1987). Alcohol may also increase the risk of successful suicide, and particular risk factors for suicide amongst alcohol abusers include adverse life events, depressed mood, physical complications and previous self-harm attempts.

Alcohol dependence is associated with a wide range of psychopathology and psychiatric problems. These can include transient intermittent auditory hallucinations, pathological jealousy, delirium tremens and secondary paranoid delusions. Delirium tremens produces an acute confusional state with disorientation in time, place and person, which can result in convulsions and has a mortality rate of 5%. The condition presents two to three days after withdrawal from alcohol, and usually remits after a week.

Alcohol misuse can lead to a deficit of vitamin B1 (thiamine), which may produce Wernike's encephalopathy, which has the characteristic triad of abnormal eye movements, staggering gait and confusion. If untreated, this can progress to Korsakoff's 'psychosis' in which the patient has a severe impairment of memory and inability to retain new information, confabulation, apathy and lack of insight.

Another chronic condition which can be caused by chronic alcohol misuse is alcoholic hallucinosis, where the patient complains of persecutory auditory hallucinations which occur in clear consciousness and with no evidence of an acute confusional state, and which may be difficult to distinguish from schizophrenia. It may occur during a period of abstinence, reduction or continued consumption of alcohol. There is an absence of thought disorder or complex delusional system, no evidence of withdrawal symptoms or family history of schizophrenia.

Comorbidity: psychiatric disorders and substance use

As shown earlier in the chapter, substance use can provide a wide range of psychopathology in its own right. The next section looks at the use of substances and its relationship with psychiatric disorders such as schizophrenia, affective and anxiety disorders, personality disorders and post traumatic stress disorder.

Schizophrenia

Recent studies have shown that up to 50% of patients suffering from schizophrenia have either drug or alcohol problems (Andreasson *et al.* 1987). Both conditions lead to impairments in cognitive, interpersonal, affective and biological functions, effects which are compounded and more difficult to overcome when they present together in the same individual. Substance use may exacerbate schizophrenic symptoms and produce psychotic symptoms in their own right, with the impact of the substance use varying depending on the class of drug used, the quantity consumed, the route of administration and the state of use. Patients may show symptoms such as mania, psychosis, depression, anxiety and personality disorder symptoms. Cocaine withdrawal may appear similar to depression with low mood, suicidal ideation and psychomotor threats. Stimulants may exacerbate psychotic symptoms, increase mood lability and interfere with sleep. Cannabis use has been reported to increase delusions, hallucinations, depression and anxiety. Schizophrenic patients who misuse alcohol may be more likely to exhibit hostile behaviour, paranoid thoughts and depression than non-alcohol using patients.

Many individuals with schizophrenia report using substances to alleviate boredom, to relieve feelings of anxiety and depression, to overcome the sedating effect of prescribed medication and to counteract the negative symptoms of schizophrenia (Mueser *et al.* 1995). However, the effect is short lived and the chronic effects of these substances are detrimental to their long-term psychological well-being and prognosis of their condition. This poor outcome may be improved by a variety of psychosocial and medication interventions, but treatment of these 'dual diagnosis' patients pose significant difficulties. They require stabilisation of their schizophrenia first, before consideration of medication to treat the additional problems of substance misuse or comorbid depression. The new atypical antipsychotics have become the first choice treatment, due to their improved compliance, tolerability, efficacy in treating negative symptoms and fewer extra-pyramidal side-effects. Medication that specifically target substance use disorders are useful for detoxification, craving reduction and relief of protracted withdrawal symptoms and can be combined with treatments for schizophrenia, and may also help to reduce the negative symptoms experienced, but there is limited research evidence at present.

Anxiety disorders

Clinical and epidemiological studies have shown substantial co-occurrence between anxiety disorders and alcohol problems (Ross *et al.* 1988), and indicate that alcohol misusers are at 2–3 times the risk of suffering from an anxiety disorder. Several hypotheses were suggested to explain this association. Family members of individuals with anxiety disorders have a greater risk of alcohol problems (Noyes *et al.* 1978). The self-medication hypothesis has been popular, and in many studies patients describe using alcohol to control their phobic fears and anxiety (Bibb & Chambless 1986). However, findings regarding the sequence of onset of anxiety disorders have been inconsistent. Schneider *et al.* (1989), found that in a sample of 98 socially phobic individuals, 16 had a past history of alcohol abuse. Social phobia preceded the onset of alcohol abuse in 15 of these 16 individuals; with most reporting using alcohol to self-medicate symptoms. However, the onset of substance misuse in other anxiety disorders has been less clear. Ross *et al.* (1988) found that the onset of anxiety disorder for most of the patients in a substance misuse centre began either after (51%) or at the same time (10%) as the alcohol use. It may be that alcohol can increase clinical anxiety; especially after prolonged drinking and during withdrawal, and thus anxiety disorders such as panic disorder and generalised anxiety disorder (GAD) may be related to these situations rather than be a primary psychiatric disorder in these individuals.

Less research has looked at the association between drug misuse and anxiety disorders, and accurate diagnosis between drug-induced states and primary anxiety disorders can be difficult. Anxiety disorders may be a risk factor for the development of drug misuse and dependence; anxiety symptoms are likely to be present during chronic intoxication and withdrawal and to influence treatment and outcome. The development of structured interviews may allow some further clarification of these issues, and observation of the symptoms during a period of abstinence may be the key to appropriate diagnosis of primary anxiety disorders in this population. Myrick and Brady (1997) looked at the relationship between social phobia and cocaine dependence and found a lifetime prevalence of social phobia in these cocaine dependent individuals to be 13.9%, with the use of cocaine following the development of social phobia. They also found that the social phobic individuals were more likely to have additional psychopathology, use poly substances and were more likely to develop alcohol abuse at an earlier age. GAD is not as well studied, and further research is required to elucidate conclusions of its relationship to drug use. One of the few studies looking at this group (Massion *et al.* 1993) found that in 63 patients with GAD, 11% had a history of drug abuse.

Mood disorders

It is recognised that there is an association between alcohol misuse and mood disorders, though the relationship is complex. As mentioned earlier, alcohol can cause many mood symptoms both due to chronic use and acute withdrawals, or may be used to self-medicate primary mood disorders. Epidemiological studies have shown a higher than expected rate of bipolar disorder and major depression, although the prevalence varies from one study to another. Strakowski *et al.* (1992) studied age of onset and comorbidity in 41 consecutive admissions for first presentation of bipolar disorder and found that 24% had a comorbid diagnosis of alcohol dependence, and that the onset of substance abuse preceded the presentation of bipolar disorder by a year in the majority of patients. The co-occurrence of these conditions raises the possibility of a common underlying biological or genetic predisposition. Clinically a history of alcohol misuse predicts an unfavourable outcome for bipolar disorder (Tohen *et al.* 1994).

It has been identified that there are sex differences in the relative frequencies of primary alcoholism and primary depression, and in the family psychiatric history of alcohol probounds. Females tend to have higher rates of primary depression with secondary alcoholism (Hesselbrock *et al.* 1985) whereas males tend to have higher rates of alcoholism with secondary depression (Schuckit 1983). It is possible that alcohol misuse and depression may be different manifestations of the same underlying illness (Winokur *et al.* 1971) and that men and women may differ in the expression of this underlying illness. Depression is considered to be important in the development of alcoholism and its clinical course, and studies have shown that effective treatment for the mood disorder has a positive impact in the outcome of alcohol related disorders.

A similar picture is true for drug use disorders and mood disorder, with studies showing high prevalence rates for this comorbidity. Again, it can be hard to distinguish if psychopathology is due to the effects of the substance in question or a primary mood disorder, but it does continue to alter the course and prognosis for the patient. The comorbidity of these two conditions also varies according to the type of drug used, and the method of its action. Cocaine is a central nervous system (CNS) stimulant and is associated with high rates of mood symptoms and disorders (Weiss *et al.* 1986), both of major depression and bipolar disorder. There is some indication that chronic cocaine use causes depletion of dopamine in the CNS, which causes both cocaine craving and a depressive syndrome, and that treatment with a tricyclic antidepressant can reduce cocaine use (Gawin & Kleber 1984), although this has not been reliably replicated. Opiate use can produce or exacerbate depressive symptoms, and opiate users appear to have difficulty managing dysphoric mood states, suggesting that dysphoria may be a primary determinant of opiate drug use. Interestingly, Strain *et al.* (1991) found that when heroin dependent patients were treated with methadone on a maintenance regime, the majority of depressive symptoms reported by subjects remitted within the first week of abstinence of treatment, which may suggest that heroin rather than all opiates can produce a depressive syndrome through a combination of pharmacological and psychosocial factors.

There have been few studies to look at the use of treatment for mood disorder in the drug-using population, and no class of antidepressant has been shown to be more effective than the others. The SSRIs tend to have a better safety profile and thus are the usual first choice for the treatment of depression in this group. Studies have also failed to show that treatment of mood symptoms leads to a reduction of drug use and thus improved outcome.

Personality disorder

There is a high prevalence of comorbidity for personality disorders and substance use disorders shown consistently in epidemiological surveys and studies particularly in relation to antisocial personality disorder (APD) and borderline personality disorder (BPD). The estimation of prevalence rate varies from 44% among alcohol patients to 79% among opiate users, and many of these individuals may have more than one type of personality disorder. Bernstein and Handelsman (1995) have proposed three mechanisms to try to explain the high levels of comorbidity:

(1) that substance abuse often takes place in the context of a deviant peer

group and that antisocial behaviours are shaped and reinforced by social group norms;

(2) that substances have the potential to alter behaviour through their effects as reinforcers or conditioning agents, linking environmental and internal cues to substance use. This may explain why, for example, addicted individuals may come to suspect other addicted individuals in order to avoid being exploited themselves, and to manipulate family and friends to get financial support; and

(3) that chronic substance use may alter personality through its direct effects on brain chemistry.

Personality disorders have been found to be related to poor treatment response and outcome in patients with comorbid substance abuse, although this has mainly been addressed in patients with ASPD. It has also been found that there is an earlier onset of substance use in this group (Skodol *et al.* 1999). It is important that treatment planning can take the presence of comorbid personality disorders into account, and thus maximize the effectiveness of treatment and outcome.

Post traumatic stress disorder

Research has shown a high level of substance use disorders with people who have trauma exposure and post traumatic stress disorder (PTSD), a condition which also has high rates of medical and psychiatric complications. Many experience a wide range of psychopathology such as survivor guilt, dysphoria, suicidality, and difficulty with memory apart from that of the traumatic event and social phobia-like symptoms similar to those seen in substance misusers. They also frequently experience a profound sense of shame leading to low self-esteem. Many of the cluster group symptoms can be produced independently by substance use, both during acute and chronic use and withdrawal states, leading to difficulty in diagnosis and treatment. Substance use can alter PTSD symptom expression as shown by Bremner *et al.* (1996), who reported a worsening of PTSD symptoms with cocaine and an improvement with opiates, alcohol and marijuana in 61 male veterans receiving inpatient treatment for PTSD.

Many substance misusers have been exposed to traumatic events at an early age. Wasserman *et al.* (1992) found that 64% of cocaine misusers had been exposed to a range of types of trauma. Ellason *et al.* (1996) found that 68% of admissions to a substance abuse treatment centre reported histories of physical and sexual abuse, usually before adolescence, although not all would qualify for a formal diagnosis of PTSD. Rates of comorbidity between substance misuse and PTSD vary between 30% and 70%, with women having a lower rate than men; this is compared to a general population rate of PTSD of 9% to 12% (Breslau *et al.* 1991; Kessler *et al.* 1995).

There are several models of comorbidity, which depend on the causal paths of the exposure to traumatic events and onset of substance misuse. Traumatic exposure can occur in the absence of substance misuse and the effects in a vulnerable individual result in substance misuse. The substance use may represent a form of self-medication to the symptoms of PTSD both the positive cluster symptoms and the negative symptoms such as emotional numbing, dysphoria and isolation. Substance use may already be present when exposure to the traumatic event occurs by altering the capacity for judgement and increased risk taking, and a high number of substance users are exposed to traumatic events (Cottler *et al.* 1992). Substance misuse and exposure to trauma resulting in PTSD may occur independently, and it may be that vulnerabilities to the negative effects of trauma exposure and to the development of substance use disorders may exist in the same individual.

It has become increasingly apparent that neurotransmitter systems, such as the dopaminergic system, are involved in both substance misuse and PTSD. Acute and chronic stress exposure leads to an increase in extracellular dopamine, and the dopaminergic reward systems are involved in the reinforcing and addicting properties of stimulants (Koob 1992) and may also be involved directly or indirectly in the reinforcing properties of alcohol, opiates and cannabinoids (Prasad *et al.* 1995). Therefore, both PTSD and many forms of substance misuse share the effect of increased central dopaminergic activity.

Conclusion

There are high rates of substance misuse and other psychiatric disorders co-morbidity in both general psychiatric and specialist addiction services. This comorbidity is associated with increased levels of violence, suicide and worse outcome including frequent and prolonged inpatient episodes. It can be difficult to distinguish psychopathology caused by effects of the substance used and that produced by a comorbid disorder thus leading to difficulty in treatment planning. Increased research and improved diagnostic instruments has led to an improvement in diagnosis and awareness. In the case of severe mental illness, this has been at least in part a product of the drive for community care and exposure of patients to the risks of alcohol and drug use.

References

American Psychiatric Association (1994) *Diagnostic and Statistical Manual of Mental, Disorders,* 4th edn. American Psychiatric Press, Washington DC.
Andreasson, S., Engstrom, A., Allebeck, P. & Rydeberg, U. (1987) Cannabis and schizophrenia: A longitudinal study of Swedish conscripts. *The Lancet* 1483–1486.
Bernstein, D.P. & Handelsman, L. (1995) The neurobiology of substance abuse and personality disorders. *Neuropsychiatry of Personality Disorders.* Blackwell Science, Cambridge.
Bibb, D.L. & Chambless, D.L. (1986) Alcohol use and abuse amongst diagnosed agoraphobics. *Behavioral Research Therapy* **24**, 49–58.
Bremner, J.D., Southwick, S.M., Darnell, A. *et al.* (1996) Chronic PTSD in Vietnam combat veterans: course of illness and substance abuse. *American Journal of Psychiatry* **153**, 369–375.
Breslau, N., Davis, G.C., Andreski, P. & Peterson, E. (1991) Traumatic events and

posttraumatic stress disorder in an urban population of young adults. *Archives of General Psychiatry* **48**, 216–222.

Brown, S.A., Inaba, R.K., Gillin, C., Schuckit, M.A., Stewart, M.A. & Irwin, M.R. (1995) Alcoholism and affective disorder: clinical course of depressive symptoms. *American Journal of Psychiatry* **152**, 45–52.

Chitwood, D.M. (1985) Factors which differentiate cocaine users in treatment from non treated users. *International Journal of Addiction* **20** (3), 449–459.

Connell, P.H. (1958) *Amphetamine Psychosis*, Maudsley Monograph Number 5. Oxford University Press, London.

Cottler, L.B., Compton, W.M., Mager, D. *et al.* (1992) Post traumatic stress disorder among substance users from the general population. *American Journal of Psychiatry* **149**, 664–670.

Cregler, M. & Mark, H. (1986) Medical complications of cocaine use. *New England Journal of Medicine* **315**, 1495–1500.

Ellason, J.W., Ross, C.A., Sainton, K. & Mayran, L.W. (1996) Axis I and II comorbidity and childhood trauma history in chemical dependency. *Bulletin of the Menninger Clinic* **60**, 39–51.

Feigner, J.P., Robins, E., Guez, S.B., Woodruff, R.A., Winokur, G. & Munoz, R. (1972) Diagnostic criteria for use in psychiatric research. *Archives of General Psychiatry* **26**, 57–63.

Gawin, F.H. & Kleber, H.D. (1984) Cocaine abuse treatment: open pilot trial with desipramine and lithium carbonate. *Archives of General Psychiatry* **41**, 903–910.

Glass, I.B. & Jackson, P. (1988) Maudsley Hospital survey: prevalence of alcohol problems and other psychiatric disorders in a hospital population. *British Journal of Addiction* **83**, 1005–1011.

Grant, B.F. (1995) Co morbidity between DSM-IV drug use disorders and major depression: results of a national survey of adults. *Journal of Substance Abuse* **7** (4), 481–497.

Hasin, D., Trautman, K., Miele, G., Samet, S., Smith, M. & Endicott, J. (1996) Psychiatric Research Interview for Substance and Mental Disorders (PRISM). Reliability in substance abusers. *American Journal of Psychiatry* **153**, 1195–1201.

Hawton, K. (1987) Assessment of suicide risk. *Br. Journal of Psychiatry* **150**, 145–153.

Hesselbrock, M.N., Meyer, R.E. & Keener, J.J. (1985) Psychopathology in hospitalized alcoholics. *Archives of General Psychiatry* **42**, 1050–1055.

Kessler, R.C., McGonagle, K.A., Zhao, S. *et al.* (1994) Lifetime and 12 month prevalence of DSM-III-R psychiatric disorders in the United States. Results from the National Comorbidity Survey. *Archives of General Psychiatry* **51** (1), 8–19.

Kessler, R.C., Sonnega, A., Bromet, E. *et al.* (1995) Post traumatic stress disorder in the National Comorbidity Survey. *Archives of General Psychiatry* **52**, 1048–1060.

Koob, G.F. (1992) Drugs of abuse: anatomy, pharmacology and function of reward pathways. *Tips* **13**, 177–193.

Mason, B.J., Kocsis, J.H., Ritvo, E.C. & Cutler, R.B. (1996) A double blind, placebo controlled trial of desipramine for primary alcohol dependance stratified on the presence or absence of major depression. *Journal of the American Medical Association* **275** (10), 761–767.

Massion, A.O., Warshaw, M.G. & Keller, M.B. (1993) Quality of life and psychiatric morbidity in panic disorder and generalized anxiety disorder. *American Journal of Psychiatry* **150** (4), 600–607.

McGrath, P.J., Nunes, E.V., Stewart, J.W. *et al.* (1996) Imipramine treatment of alcoholics with primary depression: a placebo-controlled clinical trial. *Archives of General Psychiatry* **53**, 232–240.

Merikangas, K.R. & Gerlernter, C.S. (1990) Co-morbidity for alcoholism and depression. *Psychiatric Clinics of North America* **13** (4), 613–632.

Mueser, K.T., Nishith, P., Tracy, J.I., DeGirolamo, J. & Molinaro, M. (1995) Expectations and motives for substance use in schizophrenia. *Psychiatric Clinics of North America* **21** (3), 367–378.

Mueser, K.T., Yarnold, P.R., Rosenberg, S.D. *et al.* (2000) Substance use disorders in hospitalised severely mentally ill psychiatric patients: prevalence, correlates and subgroups. *Schizophrenia Bulletin* **26** (1), 179–192.

Myrick, H. & Brady, K. (1997) Comorbid social phobia and cocaine dependence. American Psychiatric Association New Research Abstracts.

Noyes, R. Jr, Clancy, J., Crowe, R., Hoenk, P.R. & Slymen, D.J. (1978) The familial prevalence of anxiety neurosis. *Archives of General Psychiatry* **37**, 173–178.

Penick, E.C., Powell, B.J., Bingham, S.F., Liskow, B.I., Miller, N.S. & Read, M.R. (1988) A comparative study of familial alcoholism. *Journal of Studies of Alcoholism* **48**, 136–146.

Powell, B.J., Penick, E., Othmer, E., Bingham, S.F. & Rice, A.S. (1982) Prevalence of additional psychiatric syndromes among male alcoholics. *Journal of Clinical Psychiatry* **43**, 404–407.

Prasad, B.M., Sorg, B.A., Ulibarri, C. *et al.* (1995) Sensitization to stress and psychostimulants. *Annals of the New York Academy of Science* **771**, 617–625.

Regier, D.A., Myers, J.K., Kramer, M. *et al.* (1984) The NIMH Epidemiological Catchment Area programme. Historical context, major objectives, and study population's characteristics. *Archives of General Psychiatry* **41** (10), 934–941.

Ross, H.E., Glaser, F.B. *et al.* (1988) The prevalence of psychiatric disorders in patients with alcohol and other drug problems. *Archives of General Psychiatry* **45**, 1023–1032.

Rounsaville, B., Anton, S., Cattoll, K., Budde, D., Prusoff, B. & Gawin, F. (1991) Psychiatric diagnosis of treatment-seeking cocaine abusers. *Archives of General Psychiatry* **48**, 43–51.

Schneider, F.R., Martin, L.Y., Liebowitz, M.R., Gorman, J.M. & Fryer, A.J. (1989) Alcohol abuse in social phobia. *Journal of Anxiety Disorders* **3**, 15–23.

Schuckit, M.A. (1983) Alcoholic patients with secondary depression. *American Journal of Psychiatry* **140**, 711–714.

Skodol, A.E., Oldham, J.M. & Gallaher, P.E. (1999) Axis II comorbidity of substance use disorders among patients referred for treatment of personality disorders. *American Journal of Psychiatry* **156** (5), 733–738.

Strain, E.C., Stitzer, M.L. & Bigelow, G.E. (1991) Early treatment time course of depressive symptoms in opiate addicts. *Journal of Nervous and Mental Disease* **179**, 215–221.

Strakowski, S.M., Tohen, M., Stoll, A.L. *et al.* (1992) Comorbidity in mania at first hospitalization. *American Journal of Psychiatry* **149**, 554–556.

Thomas, H. (1993) Psychiatric symptoms in cannabis users. *British Journal of Psychiatry* **163**, 141–149.

Tohen, M., Shulman, K. & Satlin, A. (1994) First-episode mania in late life. *American Journal of Psychiatry* **151**, 130–132.

Tohen, M., Waternaux, C.M. & Tsuang, M.T. (1990) Outcome in mania. *Archives of General Psychiatry* **47**, 1105–1111.

Wasserman, D.A., Havassy, B.E. & Boles, S.M. (1992) Traumatic events and post traumatic stress disorder in cocaine users entering private treatment. Presented at the College on Problems of Drug Dependence Annual Meeting.

Weiss, R., Mirin, S. & Griffin, M. (1994) Methodological considerations in the diagnosis of coexisting psychiatric disorders abusers. *British Journal of Addiction* **87**, 179–187.

Weiss, R., Mirin, S.M., Michael, J.L. & Sollogub, A.C. (1986) Psychopathology in chronic cocaine abusers. *American Journal of Drug and Alcohol Abuse* **12**, 17–29.

Winokur, G., Rimmer, J. & Reich, T. (1971) Alcoholism IV: is there more than one type of alcoholism? *British Journal of Psychiatry* **118**, 525–531.

Woodruff, R.A.J., Guze, S.B. *et al.* (1972) Anxiety neurosis amongst psychiatric outpatients. *Compr. Psychiat.* **13**, 165–170.

5: European Dimension of Dual Diagnosis

Fabrizio Schifano

Introduction

There is convincing evidence, at least in some European countries (Cantwell *et al.* 1999), of an increase in the diagnosis of substance-related psychiatric disorders. This may be as a result of relative shift from hypno-sedatives to hallucinogenics and stimulants misuse since the late 1990s (Griffiths & Vingoe 1997). More precisely, with the spread of HIV/AIDS (related to the sharing of syringes by drug misusers) all around Europe in the last years of the 1980s, the intravenous use of hard drugs (like heroin) is not considered 'trendy' any longer (Schifano *et al.* 1998a). The European populations, mainly opiate consumers, are much older than those who misuse stimulants and hallucinogenic drugs. Amongst European youth cultures, only those molecules which can be snorted, inhaled or ingested are considered acceptable. The new drugs consumers do not conform to the usual profile of a heroin user and are instead employed, involved in relationships and not necessarily living in deprived areas (Schifano *et al.* 1998a). Depending on which psychoactive substance is used and how it is used, the use of those substances can create four types of dually diagnosed patients (Inaba & Cohen 1997).

(1) One kind of dual diagnosis involves the person who had a clearly defined mental illness and then gets into drugs.

(2) Dual diagnosis occurs when there might have been an underlying psychiatric problem, which has not fully developed. When that person started to use psychoactive drugs, the effects and interactions of those substances uncovered the underlying mental disturbance.

(3) Dual diagnosis occurs when the drug itself (or withdrawal from the drug) causes a transient depression, temporary psychosis, or another mental illness.

(4) Dual diagnosis happens when there was not a pre-existing problem but as a result of years of use or some reaction to the drug, the user develops a chronic psychiatric problem because the toxic effects of the drug permanently imbalance the brain chemistry.

In this chapter, an attempt is made to describe both the European trends of the drug scenario and how it has altered the perception and the approach of dual diagnosis patients in the health service treatment centres across the continent. A brief European literature is presented and some suggestions about the differences between mental health and chemical dependency treatment communities (especially with respect to what happens in some European Countries) are emphasised.

Dual diagnosis and modification of the European drug scenario

The European increase in the use of drugs with hallucinogenic (LSD, high potency cannabinols like skunk, ecstasy, ketamine, etc.) and stimulant (amphetamines, cocaine, the latter particularly in its smokeable form) properties and even poly-drug use (Parker 1997) is becoming a public health problem. In fact, in three of the four kinds of quoted dual diagnosis types, the chemical and toxicological characteristics of the drug itself are essential in determining the appearance of the mental health problems. For instance, the use of high potency cannabinols and of LSD can clearly uncover an underlying psychiatric problem in a particular patient; a temporary paranoid psychosis can be caused by cocaine intoxication. In addition, the permanent neurodegenerative effects on the side of the 5-HT2 brain neurons (McCann *et al.* 1998) could be the explanation of the appearance of several psychiatric symptoms observable in chronic MDMA (ecstasy) users (Thomasius *et al.* 1997; Schifano *et al.* 1998b).

It has been suggested (Henry 1992) that it will take many years to fully understand the real contribution of MDMA use to the onset of psychiatric disturbances. On the other hand, opiates can have a sort of 'protective' effect against the emergence of serious psychiatric problems (like psychosis) in at least some patients. In fact, our group examined the characteristics and the possible psychopathological consequences of ecstasy use in 150 consecutive patients presenting to the Padova Addiction Treatment Unit (ATU), Italy, who had taken ecstasy on at least one occasion (but 95% of them had experimented with another drug of abuse at least once in their lifetime).

Of the total sample, 53% were found to have one or more psychopathological problems. The most frequent were depression, psychotic disorders, cognitive disturbances, bulimic episodes, impulse control disorders, panic disorders, and social phobia. Those who were free from any psychopathological problem, compared to the others, had taken a smaller number of MDMA tablets in their lifetime, for a shorter duration and with a lower frequency. This particular sample were less likely to have used alcohol together with ecstasy but more likely to have used opiates. Opiate consumers were, compared to non-consumers, less likely to show psychopathological disturbances (odds ratio 0.2). From the clinical point of view, one could conclude that the use of opiates might well have masked the possible presentation of the psychiatric symptomatology of MDMA consumers. On the other hand, it is a common clinical observation that opiates (including methadone) can show appreciable therapeutic effects in controlling the psychiatric manifestations characteristic of some patients and that it is possible to observe, during the methadone tapering, the emergence of a psychotic episode.

Dual diagnosis in Europe

In many European countries, the growth of licensed professionals working in the field of substance misuse has resulted in a greater recognition and treatment of dual diagnosis patients (Inaba & Cohen 1997). In order to assess health and social care professionals working in the European Addiction Treatment Units (ATUs), issues related to dual diagnosis patients and the commonalities and differences between a cluster of European specialised drug abuse treatment centres, an examination of a transnational study (Ghodse *et al.* 1998) was undertaken. The main purpose of this transnational study was to describe the process and structure of methadone substitution therapy (MST) across Europe and the objective included an examination of individual and aggregate MST variables comprising external factors (i.e. national policy on prescribing), programme attributes (including the personnel profile) and treatment practices (i.e. type of treatment contract, dosing policy, etc.). The study was carried out in 11 ATUs across nine European countries.

The centres were chosen on the basis of their long tenure in the programme and expertise with the clinical issues. The group were members of the European Collaborating Centres in Addiction Studies (ECCAS). There were many difficulties and problems of conducting transnational studies, including language barriers, cultural, historical and political differences. Data collection was made (over a period of 24 months during 1995 and 1997) through a self-administered postal questionnaire and a semistructured interview conducted during site visits by the study co-ordinator. For the purpose of the present paper, the characteristics of the 11 ATUs' staff have been thoroughly evaluated. Out of the 279 professionals (medical doctors, psychologists, social workers, educators, drug counsellors, occupational therapists, nurses) working in the centres examined, 73 (23% of the total staff) were psychologists ($n=34$) and psychiatrists ($n=35$). This group had formal training in substance misuse and clinical experience in dual diagnosis. However, this should be regarded as a conservative estimate, since in some countries (i.e. the UK) some of the nurses and drug counsellors had had significant clinical experience in working with dual diagnosis patients. It is estimated that at least one in four professionals, all across Europe, holds clinical expertise in the recognition and management of dual diagnosis patients.

The incidence of dual diagnosis among compulsive drug users and particularly among the homeless (Vazquez *et al.* 1997; Fichter & Quadflieg 1999) remains extremely high in Europe. The contributing factors include: the diminishing number of mental health facilities (for example, see the 1978 Italian Psychiatric Reform no.180); the cutting of mental health budgets (as has happened in different European countries in recent years); the increased number of patients on prescribed medications such as antidepressants or antipsychotics and the increased reliance on outpatients mental health facilities which have forced many psychiatric patients to deal with their problems on an outpatient basis or on their own. Detached from the structure and intense professional supervision of hospital care, poor control of their prescribed medication and aggravation of mental problems are more likely to lead patients to turn to street drugs for help (Inaba & Cohen 1997).

Dual diagnosis: the European studies

A review of the literature published between 1 January 1990 and 31 December 1999 revealed that during this period, 28 papers were published in international refereed journals, 18 in America and 10 in Europe (3 from the UK, 3 from Germany and the others from Greece, Spain, Finland and Iceland). In Table 5.1, the main goals and results of these 10 relevant papers are summarised. Most of them emphasise the epidemiological importance of the issue of dual diagnosis.

The findings show that between 60% and 90% of substance misusers who are in treatment suffer from at least one psychopathological trouble and 20–50% of the patients treated by mental health services are diagnosable with a substance-related disorder. In some at-risk samples, such as homeless people, these figures are much more worrying. On the whole, clinical and social outcomes have been reported to be worse in the dual diagnosis patients and service costs greater than in individuals with severe mental illness only.

Mental health treatment community vs. chemical dependency treatment community: the Italian experience

There are several differences between the mental health and the chemical dependency treatment community centres in most European countries. In this chapter only the Italian experience is presented.

In Italy, there are about 540 Public Health Addiction Treatment Units (at least one for each Local Health Unit) which are attended each year by about 120 000 drug addicts. Most (around 85–90%) of them are opiate addicts and approximately 55 000 of them are provided with methadone on a daily basis. In some regions (like Venetia) most of the doctors working in the ATUs hold a qualification in psychiatry, whereas this is less common in other regions (like Lombardy). However, in virtually all of the Italian ATUs there is at least one clinical psychologist.

In each Local Health Unit in Italy there is at least one 15-bed psychiatric ward and one outpatient mental health treatment centre. Most of the patients attending the facilities have severe mental illnesses (bipolar disorders; schizophrenia) and, since 1978, with the Psychiatric Reform no. 180) all of the long-term psychiatric hospitals have been closed and the patients

Table 5.1 Summary of main goals and results of eight papers from Europe on the issue of dual diagnosis

Authors and country	Main goal(s) of the study	Main results
Alaja et al. (1998); Finland	To assess comorbidity of substance use disorders with physical and mental disorders among 1249 consecutive psychiatric patients admitted to six general hospitals	Over 70% of pure alcoholics and over 90% of poly-substance users had comorbid diagnoses (affective disorders were – 33% of the sample – the most prevalent)
Cantwell et al. (1999); UK	To identify the prevalence and pattern of substance and misuse in first-episode psychosis	One-year prevalence rates were 19.5% for drug misuse and 11.7% for alcohol abuse; 8.4% of the Ss received a primary diagnosis of substance-related psychotic disorder, a significant increase compared with an earlier cohort from the same catchment area
Fichter and Quadflieg (1999); Germany	To assess alcohol abuse and dependence as well as other mental disorders in a sample of homeless men	Lifetime prevalence of Axis I DSM-IV disorders was 79.6%
Gafoor and Rassool (1998); UK	Examination of the nature and extent of dual diagnosis	Discussion of the implication for mental health nurses of the dual diagnosis issues and of treatment strategies
Kokkevi et al. (1998); Greece	To assess at intake 226 drug addicts admitted in 3 major therapeutic programs	Personality disorders prevalence was 59.5%: Ss with a personality disorder were at risk of having a comorbid Axis I disorder
Krausz et al. (1999); Germany	To investigate, through 3 repeated interviews, 219 opiate addicts for the presence of mental symptoms	One third of the patients were in good mental condition in three stages, 17% worsened their psychiatric suffering whereas for another 17% their mental condition improved. There was not a marked correlation between the extent of drug consumption and mental disorders
Thomasius et al. (1997); Germany	To assess 171 Ss with psychiatric illnesses who had contact with the NHS services for their possible drug abuse	The one-year prevalence rate for any substance problem was 36.3%. Patients with dual diagnosis had spent significantly longer periods in hospital than the others
Vazquez et al. (1997); Spain	To describe the lifetime and 12-month prevalence rate of DSM-III-R mental disorders among 261 homeless Ss in Madrid	Fifty per cent of the sample had substance-related disorders; lifetime prevalence of schizophrenia was 4%

62

discharged into the community. There is an inherent difficulty in obtaining reliable data in terms of service utilisation and admissions of patients with dual diagnosis. However, in the Venetia region (one of the 20 Italian regions) there are 38 Local Health Units and around 50 psychiatric wards (with the mental health outpatient treatment centres). On the whole, Italian substance misuse treatment facilities are usually reluctant to treat dual diagnosis patients because they see them as too disruptive. Psychiatric treatment centres also avoid these patients because they are perceived as always relapsing and too chaotic to manage.

Also, in Italy, where the highest number of rehabilitative therapeutic facilities is found, there are some differences between the mental health treatment community and the drug addiction treatment community. This helps us to understand why appropriate treatment for the dually diagnosed client has proven to be difficult to obtain.

• In the mental health (MH) system, limited recovery from one's problem is acceptable, whereas in the drug addiction (DA) programme, and especially in the therapeutic communities (TC), it is believed that lifetime abstinence and recovery are possible.

• The mental health system, which has a supportive philosophy, relies on medication to help the patient, whereas DA (and especially TC) programmes promote a drug-free philosophy and use confrontation techniques. In this respect, a few of the Italian TCs have opened their doors to dual diagnosis patients, and colleagues exclusively treat this kind of drug addict. In these cases, there is a formal link with the MH local system and the medication prescription is the rule and not the exception.

• In MH, the team is exclusively composed of licensed and qualified professionals whereas in the TC professionals and former addicts very often work together.

• MH places a greater emphasis on preventing the client from getting worse, while DA programmes have some tendency to allow people to hit rock-bottom, in order to break through the denial of addiction.

Although the above statements try to summarise the different approaches in Italy, between the MH and the DA treatment communities, it seems that, to a certain extent, the situation applies equally in other European countries (such as the UK, France, Spain).

Conclusion

It is likely that the changes in the drug scenario as described may have led to an increase in diagnosis of substance-related psychiatric disorders in Europe. On the whole, it seems that the ATU professionals across Europe hold the necessary theoretical and clinical knowledge to cope with the dual diagnosis issues. In certain countries (like the UK) there are specialist dual diagnosis centres and professionals and in others (like Italy) some of the TCs specialise in adequately diagnosing and treating these patients. From the research point of view, however, most of the studies have been carried out in the USA and there has been little research in Europe (and certainly not enough, given the different patterns of substance misuse in Europe compared to America). However, interest in the field is increasing, as witnessed both by the flourishing of the sessions dedicated to the dual diagnosis issue in the most important scientific meetings and the great number of subcommittees dedicated to substance-use disorders in the different national scientific societies of psychiatry (in Italy: Società Italiana di Psichiatria; Società Italiana Comportamenti di Abuso e Dipendenza). It is hoped that in the future there will be an increase in collaboration of European professionals from mental health systems and those from addiction treatment centres so that patients will no longer be shuffled aimlessly back and forth between the two systems (Inaba & Cohen 1997) without receiving much needed health care.

References

Alaja, R., Seppa, K., Sillanaukee, P. *et al.* (1998) Physical and mental comorbidity of substance use disorders in psychiatric consultations. *European Consultation-Liaison Workgroup, Alcohol and Clinical Experimental Research* **22**, 1820–1824.

Cantwell, R., Brewin, J., Glazebrook, C. *et al.* (1999) Prevalence of substance-misuse in first-episode psychosis. *British Journal of Psychiatry* **174**, 150–153.

Fichter, M. & Quadflieg, N. (1999) Alcoholism in homeless men in the mid-nineties: results from the Bavarian Public Health Study on homelessness. *European Archives of Psychiatry and Clinical Neuroscience* **249**, 34–44.

Gafoor, M. & Rassool, G. Hussein (1998) The co-existence of psychiatric disorders and substance misuse: working with dual diagnosis patients. *Journal of Advances in Nursing* **27**, 497–502.

Ghodse, H., Clancy, C. & Oyefeso, A., eds (1998) *Methadone Substitution Therapy in Europe.* Centre for Addiction Studies, St George's Hospital Medical School, London.

Griffiths, P. & Vingoe, L. (1997) *The Use of Amphetamines, Ecstasy and LSD in the European Community: A Review of Data on Consumption Patterns and Current Epidemiological Literature.* Report prepared for the European Monitoring Centre for Drugs and Drug Abuse (EMCDDA), London.

Henry, J. (1992) Ecstasy and the dance of death. *British Medical Journal* **305**, 5–6.

Inaba, D. & Cohen, S., eds (1997) Eccitanti, sedativi, psichedelici. Piccin Nuova Libraria, Padua.

Kokkevi, A., Stefanis, N., Anastasopoulou, E. & Kostogianni, C. (1998) Personality disorders in drug abusers: prevalence and their association with Axis I disorders as predictors of treatment retention. *Addict Behavior* **23**, 841–853.

Krausz, M., Verthein, U. & Degkwitz, P. (1999) Psychiatric comorbidity in opiate addicts. *European Addict Research* **5**, 55–62.

McCann, U.D., Szabo, Z., Scheffel, U., Dannals, R.F. & Ricaurte, G. (1998) Positron emission tomographic evidence of toxic effects of MDMA ('Ecstasy') on brain serotonin neurons. *The Lancet* **352**, 1433–1437.

Menezes, P.R., Johnson, S., Thornicroft, G., Marshall, J., Prosser, D., Bebbington, P. & Kuipers, E. (1996) Drug and alcohol problems among individuals with severe mental illness in south London. *British Journal of Psychiatry* **168**, 612–619.

Parker, H. (1997) L.S.D., amphetamines and ecstasy use in Europe and the research agenda. In: P. Griffiths & L. Vingoe (eds) *The Use of Amphetamines, Ecstasy and LSD in the European Community: A Review of Data on Consumption Patterns and Current Epidemiological Literature.* Report prepared for the EMCDDA, London, pp. 29–33.

Schifano, F., Corazza, O. & Forza, G. (1998a) Le sostanze d'abuso del sabato sera. In: R. Gatti (ed.) *Ecstasy E Nuove Droghe.* F. Angeli Editore, Milan, pp. 122–141.

Schifano, F., Forza, G., Di Furia, L., Minicuci, N. & Bricolo, R. (1998b) MDMA ('ecstasy') consumption in the context of poly-drug abuse: a report on 150 patients. *Drug and Alcohol Dependency* **52**, 85–90.

Thomasius, R.R., Schmolke, R. & Kraus, D. (1997) MDMA ('ecstasy') use: an overview of psychiatric and medical sequelae. *Fortschitte der Neurologogie Psychiatrie* **65**, 49–61.

Tomasson, K. & Vaglum, P. (1995) A nationwide representative sample of treatment seeking alcoholics: a study of psychiatric comorbidity. *Acta Psychiatrica Scandinavia* **92**, 378–385.

Vazquez, C., Munoz, M. & Sanz, J. (1997) Lifetime and 12-month prevalence of DSM-III-R mental disorders among the homeless in Madrid: a European study using the CIDI. *Acta Psychiatrica Scandinavia* **95**, 523–530.

6: Misperceiving Complex Behaviour: A Psychological Research Model

Fred Roach

Introduction

In recent times, there has been an increase in the interest in dual diagnosis and the literature is expanding. However, there is still an apparent dearth in the history of the nosology of dual diagnosis and a nosography does not, so far, exist. This is not at all surprising because the label has now become less meaningful in clinical practice. In classical presentations, the stages of an illness, disease or disorder are described along with explanations of its origins, prodromes, symptoms, prognosis and complications. The same can not be said in the case of dual diagnosis.

In psychiatry generally, every cluster of syndromes was dealt with in a classical way and all the perceived conditions were gradually arranged in a traditional order. However, attempts at subdividing these groups of syndromes into specific types of a particular mental illness or personality disorder were later discouraged because of the emergence of some apparent instabilities within and between syndromic groups. This observation signalled the difficulty posed by the use of the medical model to describe complex behaviour profiles. It also pointed to the recognition that individuals' complex behaviour can not be explained merely in terms of ascribed psychiatric labels.

The apparent postclassical return to identifying core psychiatric pathology as a basis for labelling psychiatric illness or personality disorder and establishing a nosology, has brought the problem of dual diagnosis into focus. Although the concept is reasonable, the label is now so loosely and homogenously applied by clinicians and non-clinicians alike, that its value in establishing meaningful debate on the nature of the comorbidity in the affected individual, is questionable. Generally, the current use of the term offers no universal explanation of the nature of the comorbidity condition, or problem, affecting the individual to whom it is applied. Neither does it provide a clear direction for guiding those who are tasked with the responsibility of helping the individual who presents with the dual diagnosis label.

In the light of recent reviews (e.g. Mental Health Act; National Service Framework for Mental Health) this chapter offers a contribution to the growing debate on dual diagnosis. It presents some preliminary findings from part of an ongoing longitudinal study which commenced in August 1998, on a cohort of patients with complex behaviour profiles who were labelled as dual diagnosis patients. This selection of patients was admitted to a forensic setting for assessment, treatment and rehabilitation. They were perceived as requiring a secure environment because of public concern, as well as their dangerousness and risk of self-harm and harm to others. The prime aim was to apply a psychological research model to the investigation of this group of dual diagnosis patients to attempt to identify the main and subordinate characteristics of their complex behaviour and to investigate the presence of certain psychological and behavioural factors that characterise their complex behaviour profile and to assess any change in the complexity of the profile over time.

Complex behaviour

Behaviour can be perceived in terms of a continuum, from simple to complex, which forms a normal distribution curve. In the context of psychological medicine, complex behaviour refers to behaviour which contains a main characteristic (e.g. psychiatric illness or personality disorder, learning disabilities, alcohol or substance misuse, physical condition, forensic history, psychological or behavioural, etc.) and one or more subordinate characteristics with one or more intra- or interrelated features (e.g. aggression, violence, self-harm, arson, sexual abuse, etc.). Psychologically, complex behaviour is dangerous behaviour; its impact upon the affected individual and colleagues with whom the individual comes into contact should not be under-estimated. Nor should complex behaviour be judged synonymously with complex needs. The needs are not dangerous, it is the behaviour that is dangerous. The needs are profound.

Psychiatrists, and other clinicians, who are presented with complex behaviour are dealing with individuals who are functioning at the extremes of a normal distribution. It must be acknowledged therefore that there will be some discontinuities in the presentation of some features of the main characteristic of the complex behaviour, as officially categorised (e.g. ICD-10, WHO 1992; DSM-1V, APA 1994) as well as discontinuities in subordinate characteristics, in different individuals, over time. There is therefore a danger in treating specific discontinuities, either in the main or subordinate characteristics of the complex behaviour profile, as independent conditions, as implied by the attachment of the label 'dual diagnosis'. The label assumes the presence of two distinct diagnoses, whereas in the context of complex behaviour, the individual may have a number of concurrent subordinate problems or difficulties apart from one main problem which attracts a diagnosis. Recent use of the term, among professionals and lay persons alike, has thus reactivated both the classification problem in psychiatry and issues around the application of the medical model to psychological medicine.

Some theoretical and clinical issues

Theoretical and clinical explanations of the dual diagnosis phenomenon have so far tended to focus on the identification of psychiatric features as main characteristics associated with psychiatric illness or personality disorder, alcohol and substance misuse, etc. Attempts are then made at discriminating among perceived psychiatric illnesses or personality disorders or other conditions and pairing any perceived differentiation with subordinate characteristics associated with offending, maladaptive, or social behaviour problems and assigning the dual diagnosis label to the individual. This approach has relied on the medical model for its perception, conceptualisation and representation of complex behaviour. Such strong attachment to the use of the medical model in this context and for the subsequent implementation of risk management strategies to deal with those affected, has not been without criticism (Russell 1993). It is the author's view that complex behaviour needs to be explored in ways other than by an approach which results in a dual diagnosis labelling of the affected individual. The use of the term 'dual diagnosis' as a way of packaging psychiatric illness or personality disorder, with offending, maladaptive, or social behaviour problems, as a single co-morbidity diagnosis concept, amounts to the possible misperception and medicalisation of complex behaviour.

The idea that people may present a problem in different ways, or in ways which may match criteria associated with more than one morbidity, at the same time, is not new. For many years, psychiatry has witnessed a lack of consensus in the establishment of some clinical judgements, formulation of diagnosis and in ascribing psychiatric labels to known features of main or subordinate characteristics (e.g. mental illness or alcohol and substance misuse) of complex behaviour. It is known that not all psychiatrists would classify the same presenting problem, or set of problems, in the same way (Kreitman *et al.* 1961; Zublin 1967). Also, the same patient may be judged differently by different psychiatrists, despite similar orientation and training. Transculturally, it is also not unknown for the same person to present problems differently to different people and still be misunderstood. The literature shows that this particular misunderstanding may have led to over-representation among compulsory admissions of Afro-Caribbeans and Asians to psychiatric hospitals (Pinsent 1963; Kiev 1965; Littlewood & Lipsedge 1981; Harrison *et al.* 1984; Littlewood 1988), to a longer stay in hospital than their white counterparts and to higher doses of antipsychotic medication being administered. This has been apparent even where side-effects to drugs might be severe, or where the drug might, in some cases, precipitate the onset of a serious physical disability.

Historically, disagreements on nomenclature have been echoed (Ash 1949; Hunt *et al.* 1953; Schmidt & Fonda 1956; Kreitman 1961; Beck 1962; Ward *et al.* 1962, 1964). A questioning of the use of the label 'dual diagnosis' was noted in the early nineteenth century, when Georget posited the view that there was only one psychosis which was organic in cause but had many different forms. Later, Kraepelin (1909–13) placed emphasis on the course of the illness in the development of a classification system. It seems apparent from this history that universal consensus on the use and understanding of dual diagnosis can not be assumed. What the label conveys to one person, including the patient, may be quite different from what it conveys to another. It is likely that the term has become yet another way of ascribing powerful psychiatric labels to individuals whose complex behaviour is difficult to interpret, differentiate or formulate in terms of a single diagnostic category. One such example is the label 'ganja-psychosis' which emerged as a form of dual diagnosis for Afro-Caribbeans with mental illness who also had an alcohol or substance misuse problem or forensic history and a culturally related social behaviour problem (Cochrane 1977; Carpenter & Brockington 1980; London 1986; McGovern & Cope 1987; Harrison *et al.* 1988; Roach 1992).

Psychological research model

The apparent confusion which surrounds the labelling of people as dual diagnosis strengthens the call for the application of a psychological research model to investigate the characteristics of complex behaviour, in particular in cases where the medical model might be limited. It is acknowledged that some inferences may be drawn from psychiatric symptomatology (Maxwell 1973). However, the early attachment of a dual diagnosis label to an individual without a detailed investigation of the psychological and behavioural factors that characterise the complex behaviour profile, is not recommended. In the writer's opinion, these factors should not be examined as if 'in a box' from which existing psychiatric labels (e.g. ICD-10, WHO 1992; DSM-1 V, APA 1994) could be withdrawn and simply attached to the individual. Such allocated labels do tend to become the medium through which all further communication with the individual is conducted and to which observers respond, with risk management and other strategies.

The psychological research model seems the most appropriate way forward to investigate the existence of psychological and behavioural factors in an individual's complex behaviour profile. In the context of the main and subordinate characteristics that are present in the individual's complex behaviour, the manifestation of psychiatric features may form only one part of the observed complexity rather than evidence of the whole condition that merit being labelled dual diagnosis. A psychological research model, which adopts a systematic approach to the investigation of human behaviour, may assist in the detection of assets or deficits among factors which may influence the manifestation of psychiatric illness or personality disorder, alcohol or substance misuse problems, or a social behaviour problem, to which specific psychiatric labelling may or may not be rationally applied, or to which the individual's complex behaviour can or can not be fully attributed.

Intra- and inter-factor integration

Many psychological, behavioural and social factors are responsible for the manifestation of complex behaviour in the individual. The dynamic integration of these factors in the individual's intra- and interphysical, biological and psychological disposition is acknowledged. Anthropological influences on intra- or inter-factors, the person's socialisation, personal experiences, life events, significant others and definition of the situation all play a part. Thus, the main or subordinate characteristic of the complex behaviour that is brought to the attention of others may be driven by one, or any combination of, these variables. The stability or instability of the main characteristic itself may subsequently be determined by the intra- and interrelationship of the individual's body and mind. A psychological research model would, in the author's view, assist in systematically exploring an individual's psychobiological makeup and experience of the world and allow some identification of the role that the dynamic organisation of the inter- and intra-factors play in determining the complex behaviour profile. A sense of multifacetedness, with the individual functioning as a whole while displaying different elements of dysfunction within their complex behaviour profile, must be the focus of perceiving and understanding complex behaviour. The notion of dual diagnosis, as currently conceptualised, seems not to take account of this position. The individual, it would seem, is perceived as being 'dual diagnosis'; and so labelled and framed.

Early twentieth century writers, such as Goffman (1968) and Parsons (1937, 1951, 1995), were detailed in their analysis of the negative effects of labels (e.g. the process of stigmatisation (Goffman) and the role of social stratification (Parsons)). More recently, Russell (1993) found that remand prisoners who were perceived as 'dual diagnosis' were less likely to receive help than those with a single diagnosis. It is also known that lay persons and professionals alike might react or respond more or less favourably to one or both labels (Russell 1993).

The danger also rests with the individual who might continually act out the ascribed labels, in terms of the sick-role (Parsons 1960), intentionally or not, for personal or secondary gain, associated with social or welfare benefit or psychological needs. Thus, individuals may engage in a process of rotating and benefiting from each element of a dual diagnosis in accordance with their perceived need at the time. This may also arise from others misperceiving complex behaviour as complex needs which may lead to an inappropriate search for ways of meeting profound needs. Wilkins's (1969) use of the term 'label-amplification', in his explanation of social deviance as a self-fulfilling prophesy, becomes applicable to this context. When the ascribed label 'dual diagnosis', is continually restated and bestowed upon the individual, it becomes the means by which the person is known and the medium through which all subsequent action related to that person is determined. The individual's self-perception of being 'dual diagnosis', or of what others might perceive of the label, or others' subjective interpretation of the dual diagnosis label, may thus have a negative effect upon therapeutic interventions, responses of the affected person or to the outcome of attempts at effecting change in the individual's complex behaviour profile. This process, which is likely to result in the reinforcement of the subordinate characteristics of the individual's complex behaviour, in the writer's opinion is best termed 'dual-diagnosis amplification'. The aim therefore must be to establish a clearer understanding of the individual's complex behaviour and to attempt to reduce, not increase, the level of societal stigmatisation.

Creating change in the individual

The interaction between personality dimensions and situational variables is seen as most important in creating change in the individual's complex behaviour profile. A number of studies have highlighted the presence of high rates of psychosocial problems among individuals with complex behaviour including family, financial, housing, self-care, etc. (Drake & Wallach 1989). The need therefore is to know how the unique psychological and behavioural factors present in the individual affect their way of responding to stress, life events, tendency to be asocial, emotional occurrences, and so on. This knowledge, which may be derived from the use of a psychological research model, may be useful in the interest of providing therapeutic intervention and meeting their profound needs.

The community principle which embraces the social learning philosophy that if social forces could produce harmful effects, it should be possible to harness them for patients' good, offers hope for effecting change in the individual's complex behaviour profile. This can be placed in the context of Russell's (1945) view that everyday influences contribute to the overall behaviour of people, the idea being that placement of the individual with complex behaviour in an environment which emphasises and actively utilises the natural social relationship that exists in the individual's social world may engender change in their behaviour, despite the individual's internal or external control tendencies (Rotter 1971).

Assumptions and hypotheses

The primary assumption is that the individual's complex behaviour is characterised by certain detectable psychological and behavioural factors. This position invites application of the psychological research model to investigate the existence of certain psychological and behavioural factors and to describe their profiling character. The objective would be to describe the detected psychological and behavioural factors associated with the individual's observed complex behaviour as an alternative to ascribing the label 'dual diagnosis' which, from the historical background, is not consistently applied to the perceived behaviour. This approach focuses on the public personality and is concerned with the description and prediction of behaviour. The psychological research model offers an opportunity to achieve a global description of an individual's complex behaviour which could be explored in terms of the likelihood of change over time. A number of hypotheses arise from the various propositions embodied within the primary assumption:

(1) That certain detectable psychological and behavioural factors do exist in patients who are labelled 'dual diagnosis' which characterise their complex behaviour.

(2) That detected psychological and behavioural factors act as determinants of the complex behaviour profile.

(3) That detected psychological and behavioural factors that characterise the complex behaviour profile of patients who are admitted to a therapeutic community setting will change over time.

Setting

The close supervision unit (CSU) which provided the setting for testing the hypotheses is managed by an NHS Trust in Surrey in the south-east of England. It was opened in December 1993. It provides a service for patients under the Mental Health Act 1983 (DHSS 1983) who require low to low–medium secure supervised care, normally involving up to six months' stay. Some admissions come via court diversion or directly from prison. Referrals for those who are physically frail; require detoxification from drugs or alcohol; have learning disabilities, or organic brain damage; or where neurological disease is the primary problem, are excluded.

The culture and philosophy of the unit are embodied within the principles and assumptions of the therapeutic community (TC) approach. These are preservation of the patient's individuality; the assumption that patients are trustworthy; that good behaviour must be encouraged; that patients must be assumed to retain the capacity for a considerable degree of responsibility and initiative; and the encouragement of therapeutic activity exercised within a proper working day's programme for all patients.

The therapeutic community approach

A full account of the literature on the therapeutic community approach is not intended here because much has been reported elsewhere — definitions, function, effectiveness, etc. (Main 1946, 1967, 1983; WHO 1953; Jones 1959; Clark 1965; Filstead & Rossi 1973; Trauser 1984; Genders & Player 1995; Knowles 1995; Schimmel 1997), to which the reader could refer. The basic idea of the approach is to utilise the interactions which arise between people living in the same environment as the means of focusing on their complex behaviour; and, to harness the social forces of the group as the medium through which changes in their behaviour can be initiated. Jones (1959) suggested that the concept implied a change in the usual status of patients who became active participants in the therapy of other patients in contrast to their relatively more passive recipient role as patients with complex behaviour in conventional treatment regimes.

It is noteworthy that no two therapeutic communities that offer help for people with complex behaviour are the same; different models exist but the principles of self-determination and the possibilities for developing self-awareness are the same in each community model. Bell and Ryan (1985) identified three basic models: first, a therapeutic community with a psycho-analytic focus; second, an activities-oriented therapeutic community that emphasises high quality biologically oriented treatment; and, third, a thera-peutic community that focuses on psychosocial rehabilitation by addressing patients' vocational, housing and social needs. It was observed that the activ-ities-oriented therapeutic community may not necessarily operate independ-ently, therefore two more distinct and different approaches were identified: first, the analytic approach where the therapists maintain a distance, observ-ing, commenting and facilitating problem solution by interpretation of the overt and latent content of the group's interactions; and second, the rehabil-itatory socio-dynamic approach where there are several therapists repre-senting different facets of community life, and where there is an emphasis on confrontation of patients' complex behaviour here and now rather than on analytic interpretation. These approaches are not mutually exclusive; a therapeutic community may, at different times, use all these processes.

It was acknowledged that others (Westreich *et al.* 1996; Taylor *et al.* 1997) have modified aspects of the TC approach for dually diagnosed patients. These principles of modern milieu therapy (Gunderson 1983) were there-fore incorporated in the rehabilitatory socio-dynamic approach which formed the basis of the CSU's specific therapeutic community approach (Fig. 6.1).

Whilst taking account of the Butler Report (Home Office 1975), the TC approach also took account of Stubblebin (1973), who suggested processes that assist in changing behaviour. These include:
• the belief that human beings are able psychologically to help one another regardless of their education, specialised knowledge or administra-tive positions
• the belief that the group's cohesiveness depends on inclusiveness
• the idea that the patient becomes more productive and able to form reasonably satisfying emotional bonds with others
• the view that authority relationships must be openly recognised and accepted.

In addition to the patient's mutual adherence to a goal plan (Horsley 1982) within an established therapeutic community core programme, the ideas of Bloor and McKegancy (1987) for promoting therapy and engaging effective ways of increasing patients' awareness of the changeability of the community structure were incorporated into each patient's individual care plan as specific needs-related activities.

Research method

A repeated measures research design involving testing and re-testing with

INDIVIDUAL
Stability of Main and/or Subordinate Characteristics of Complex Behaviour
↑

REHABILITATION
Optimal Level of Function
Adaptive Behaviours
↑

MULTI-PROFESSIONAL
|
**Medical
Nursing
Psychology
Occupational Therapy
Chaplaincy
Art Therapy
Drama Therapy
Family Therapy
Aromatherapy**

|
THERAPEUTIC INTERVENTIONS

↑

THE GROUP APPROACH
Rehabilitatory/Socio-Dynamic
↑

THERAPEUTIC COMMUNITY APPROACH
Principles and Assumptions
↑

CLOSE SUPERVISION UNIT
Secure Setting
↑

PATIENT
Complex Behaviour

Fig. 6.1 An outline of the CSU's rehabilitatory socio-dynamic therapeutic community approach

standardised psychological and other tests was used (Kirk 1982; Keppel 1991; Barker *et al.* 1995) to detect psychological and behavioural factors and assess change in patients' complex behaviour profile over time. Specific tests were routinely administered to each patient on three occasions, i.e. two, 12 and 24 weeks, after admission. Table 6.1 lists the psychological tests used for identifying certain core psychological and behavioural factors associated with the individual's complex behaviour profile.

Additional information on past behaviour was gathered by more qualitative methods (Taylor & Bosdan 1984; Good & Watts 1989; Parry 1992) from clinical interviews, historical documents and records, multi-professional ob-

Table 6.1 Psychological tests used in the repeated measures design for identifying psychological and behavioural factors associated with the individual's complex behaviour profile

Measures	Brief overview	Purpose of use
*Wechsler Adult Intelligence Scale	Revised WAIS-R, Wechler (1981)	To test overall cognitive ability
Sixteen Personality Factor Questionnaire	16PF, IPAT (1972)	To measure personality factors
Eysenck Personality Questionnaire	EPQ-R, Eysenck & Eysenck (1975)	To measure personality dimension
Rotter Internal–External Questionnaire	I-E, Rotter (1966)	To measure nature of control
General Health Questionnaire	GHQ-28, Goldberg (1978)	To measure psychiatric caseness
Hostility and Direction of Hostility Questionnaire (HDHQ)	Caine *et al.* (1967)	To measure hostility/ direction of hostility
Self-Evaluation Questionnaire	STAI-T, Spielberger (1968)	To measure State–Trait anxiety
Beck Depression Inventory	BDI, Beck *et al.* (1979)	To measure mood/affective state
*Beck Anxiety Scale	BAI, Beck *et al.* (1988)	To measure level of anxiety

The individual's performance on these psychometric measures was reported specifically to the psychological test re-test result, with accompanying norm scores. An interpretation of the results is provided, in line with current clinical psychological judgement associated with the specific test mean score, on detected psychological or behavioural factors associated with the main or subordinate characteristics in females and males complex behaviour profile.
*These measures were only administered for initial test data.

scrvational assessments and reports. Patients' personal accounts of their life experiences and self-perception (Preston & Vinev 1984) were also acknowledged. An established set of rating scales was also used to assess the patient's current level of social functioning and assist setting targets as a further means of evaluating change (Perkins & Russell 1988; Perkins 1994; Santana *et al.* 1997). These included Health of the Nation Outcome Scale (HoNOS) (HMSO 1992) to measure degree of disability; Liverpool University Neuroleptic Side-effects Rating Scale (LUNSERS) (Day *et al.* 1995) to measure response to chemotherapy; and the Lancashire Quality of Life Profile (LQOLP) to measure quality of life/satisfaction. The combination of the findings from these quantitative and qualitative measures assisted in developing an individual care plan (ICP) and assessing change in patients' complex behaviour profile over time.

Subjects

A cohort of 26 patients were admitted to the CSU over the first two years (1998–2000) of the ongoing study. Only the subjects for the first year of study are presented here. These consisted of 13 patients—8 males and 5 females (62% and 38% of subjects, respectively) whose average age was 30 years with a range between 18 and 51 years. Most were educated beyond the age of 16 years but (38%) went to a special school due to their complex behaviour. One (male) patient had progressed to further education but failed to complete the course because of the severity of complex behaviour characteristics (i.e. his mental illness, drug abuse and maladaptive behaviour). Of the cohort, 92% had only ever had casual employment and all were unemployed at the time of admission. Forty-six per cent came from broken homes and 15% had been sexually abused.

Results

Complex behaviour profile: main and subordinate characteristics

The subjects who informed this report consisted of 13 patients (8 males and 5 females), with complex behaviour profiles. The main characteristic of the complex behaviour was identified by a psychiatric label as mental illness or personality disorder. A further label, that attracted the comorbidity, fell within the subordinate characteristics of the behaviour. Table 6.2 outlines the main and subordinate characteristics of the complex behaviour profiles of this patient group.

The outline shows that this was a group with a varied mixture of main and subordinate behaviour characteristics which constituted the complex behaviour profile. Each patient had one main characteristic or labelled diagnosis, e.g. schizophrenia, schizo-affective disorder, bipolar affective disorder or personality disorder, and one other subordinate characteristic, labelled diagnosis, e.g. alcohol or drugs misuse, which was associated with their comorbidity status plus evidence of forensic or offending behaviour, maladaptive behaviour and detached or atypical social behaviour. These were associated with personal histories of dangerousness, self-harm, aggression, violence, arson, actual and or grievous bodily harm, theft, sexual abuse and other deviant behaviours, which made up the unique complex behaviour profile.

The majority of patients (85%) had a drug or alcohol problem, or were poly-drug users. There was one case of Asperger's Syndrome (i.e. severe and sustained impairment in social interaction and the development of restricted, repetitive patterns of behaviour, interests and activities) who also had epilepsy in combination with learning disabilities. Two female patients (15%) had a diagnosis of epilepsy; two patients (one male and one female; 15%) were described as having learning disabilities and one patient (female; 8%) was diabetic. All 13 patients were detained under the Mental Health Act (1983). Eight patients (six males, two females; 62%) had an index offence, one male was on licence from prison. Five patients (two males, three females; 38%) had committed serious offences but had never been charged because of lack of sufficient evidence, or lack of motivation on the part of vic-

Table 6.2 An outline of the main and subordinate characteristics of the complex behaviour profiles of the dually diagnosed patients

Patient no.	Main characteristic	Subordinate characteristics		Maladaptive behaviours	
	Diagnosis	Diagnosis	Forensic/offending behaviour	Antisocial/asocial	Social
1*	Schizo-affective disorder	Asperger's syndrome + epilepsy	ABH, sexual	Aggression and irresponsible shopping	Detached/atypical
2▲	Personality disorder	Drug/alcohol abuse	GBH	Violence and aggression	Detached/atypical
3▲	Depression	Learning disability + drug/alcohol use	Arson	Aggression, malicious damage to property	Detached/atypical
4*	Schizo-affective disorder	Drug/alcohol abuse	Arson	Violence and aggression	Detached/atypical
5*	Schizophrenia	Diabetes + alcohol use	ABH	Aggression, shop-lifting	Detached/atypical
6*	Borderline personality disorder	Drug/alcohol abuse	None	Aggression, self-harm	Detached/atypical
7▲	Paranoid schizophrenia	Drug/alcohol abuse	ABH	Dangerous behaviours, e.g. self-neglect, violent threats	Detached/atypical
8▲	Schizophrenia	Excessive alcohol use	None	Dangerous behaviours, e.g. para-suicide, homicide threats	Detached/atypical
9*	Personality disorder	Epilepsy	None	Self-harm	Detached/atypical
10▲	Schizophrenia	Drug abuse	GBH, theft	Violence, aggression, deception	Detached/atypical
11▲	Personality disorder	Drug/alcohol abuse	Car theft + driving offences	Aggression, violence	Detached/atypical
12▲	Bipolar disorder	Alcohol dependence	Rape	Threats of violence, aggression and homicide	Detached/atypical
13▲	Personality disorder	Drug/alcohol abuse	ABH	Aggression, violence	Detached/atypical

Gender: ▲ male, * female.

tims, to progress the case through the criminal justice system. These findings suggest that the term dual diagnosis does not fully embrace an individual's complex behaviour profile. The label might prove useful as a means of focusing minds on the dynamic integration of acquired and inherited psychological or behavioural aetiological factors in relation to the main and subordinate characteristic of an individual's behaviour although it remains limited in respect of understanding the total makeup of that individual's complex behaviour profile.

Psychological and behavioural factors

Data were derived from test and from testing and re-testing of individuals from a battery of psychological tests over time. These are presented in Table 6.3.

Initial test data

The WAIS-*R*-test data showed that the patient group's ($N = 13$) overall mean Full IQ was 87.33. This indicated that this cohort of patients fell within the low average intelligence range. Females ($N = 5$) performed better than males ($N = 8$) on this test, showing an average overall intellectual capacity [i.e. F = 90.8, M = 84.86]. Men were a low average ability group. This trend was

Table 6.3 Patient group test and test re-test data from battery of psychological tests

Psychometric assessments	Mean scores at time 1 ($N=13$)	Mean scores at time 2 ($N=9$)	Mean scores at time 3 ($N=6$)	Norm scores
WAIS- R Overall IQ	87.33			Average: 90–99
WAIS-R Perform. IQ	82.92			
WAIS-R Verbal IQ	89.17			
BAI	22.62			7.78; s.d. 5.65
BDI	21.77	20.11	25	10.90; s.d. 8.10
STAI-S	48.15	51.67	53.5	F=35.12, s.d. 9.25 M=36.35, s.d. 9.67
STAI-T	52.17	50.08	56.83	F=38.25, s.d. 9.14 M=37.68, s.d. 9.69
Rotter's I–E Scale	12.08	15.5	11.5	Medium +/−11.5
EPQ-R Psychoticism	12.62	12.43		F=5.73, s.d. 3.85 M=7.19, s.d. 4.60.
EPQ-R Extraversion	15.08	12		F=14.14, s.d. 5.06 M=12.51, s.d. 6.00
EPQ-R Neuroticism	15.69	16.14		F=12.47, s.d. 5.22 M=10.54, s.d. 5.81.
EPQ-R Lie scale	8.38	9		F=6.88, s.d. 3.97 M=7.10, s.d. 4.28.
EPQ-R Addiction	16.46	16.43		F=12.61, s.d. 4.18 M=11.60, s.d. 4.96.
EPQ-R Criminality	18.77	17.29		Controls=9.01, s.d. 4.54 Prisoners=15.57, s.d. 5.18.
GHQ-28	11.31	11.6	12.66	Threshold=5
HDHQ-Hostility	28	26.56	31.83	13.0, s.d. 6.2
HDHQ-Direction of Hostility	−3.85	−1.11	0.67	+0.5, s.d. 4.6

Note: It was not possible to complete the WAIS assessment with one male patient, therefore for the WAIS assessment, all patients $N=12$, males $N=7$, females $N=5$.

also reflected in the verbal and performance IQ subscales where male verbal skills reflected a borderline ability. Generally, this was a group of patients who were aware of what they were doing and could be held responsible for their behaviour. It could be said that females were more premeditated in their actions than were males and showed more in-depth understanding of their current situation. Females were more able to verbalise their problems than were the males who were more likely to act out aspects of their complex behaviour profile without prior acknowledgement of the consequences.

The BAI generated test data for anxiety. The mean score was 22.62 which represented a picture of moderate anxiety for this patient group. When the mean score for males ($N = 8$) 18.25 was separated from the mean score for females ($N = 5$) 29.60, it showed that the females were more likely than males to reflect a generalised state of anxiety.

In general, the results from the tests on patients' ability and on their tendency towards situational anxiety suggest some assumed potential influence over the identified main and subordinate characteristics of their complex behaviour profile.

Repeated measures data

The test and re-test measures investigated any fundamental change in the complex behaviour profile over time. It was acknowledged that patients admitted under the CSU criteria would normally be expected to remain on the unit for a period of six months. However, due to the complexity of the patients' behaviour profile and to the rehabilitatory nature of its therapeutic community approach, it would be unlikely that all patients would fulfil this criteria (54% of the 13 patients remained for six months, or longer). One male patient (8%) remained too psychotic for further testing over time. Only 46% of the patient group fully completed the test and re-test measures.

The mean score on general health was above the threshold of 5 at the time of the first assessment, within the first two weeks of admission (T1) and remained high over time. This suggested 'psychiatric caseness' among this group. Both males and females, had enduring mental illness or personality disorder which needed attention but females had far more severe psychiatric problems than the males. These patients required help for their main and subordinate behaviour characteristics, in terms of comorbidity, at the time of admission and beyond.

Mean scores for depression represented a picture of a group that was affected by moderately low mood, over time. When the mean score for males was separated from the mean score for females, it showed that the females were more severely affected and were more likely to remain in this state over time, than men.

The mean scores for State/Trait Anxiety were well above the range for normal subjects. These scores are representative of dually diagnosed patients who manifest anxiety as part of their pathological personality associated with an enduring mental illness reflected by depression, generalised anxiety and schizophrenia complicated by brain damage and character disorder. Females were more likely to show an underlying state of anxiety as part of their normal and/or pathological personality than were the males. These means remained well above the range for normal subjects over time. The results confirmed some stability in the underlying STAI-T factors. Females remained in a severe state of anxiety whereas, males remained minimally to moderately anxious.

The mean score for internal–external control was 12.08. This score fell within the external domain and reflected a group of patients who felt that their fates were in the hands of powerful others, or externally controlled. As a group, they felt that they did not control themselves or their destinies. Females were far more inclined to feel externally controlled than were males who felt no more internally than externally controlled.

The mean score for hostility and direction of hostility was 28 and −3.85, respectively. These scores suggested that this was a very hostile group of individuals who had a history of violence associated with their mental health state. They would tend to express resistance through violence or aggression on people or property. When the mean score for males was separated from the mean score for females, it showed that the females were far more hostile than were the males. However, the direction of hostility was more external for males than for females who tended to be more intropunitive. The hostility and direction of hostility remained stable in both males and females, over time.

The mean scores for Eysenck's personality dimensions of psychoticism, extraversion and neuroticism were calculated. For psychoticism the total mean score was above the average for males, and for females. This reflected a group of individuals with some underlying personality variables which could be associated with an enduring mental illness or personality disorder. This group tend to be solitary, not caring for people, often troublesome, not fitting in anywhere. This was a group that may be cruel and inhumane, lacking in feeling and empathy, and altogether insensitive. There is hostility to others and violence or aggression, even to loved ones. The females in this group were just as likely as the males to reject change and show no guilt feelings, empathy or sensitivity to others.

The mean score for extraversion was within the average range for males and females. The nature of this group's social interaction was at a level which would normally be expected, but females were less inclined to engage socially than were males. The mean score for neuroticism was within the average range for males and females. This was a group of patients who do not worry too much about what they do. Females were no more inclined towards high levels of neurotic behaviours than were the males in this group.

The mean scores on three additional scales on the EPQ-R showed the following: for addiction the mean score fell within the average range for normals among the males, but above the average for normals among the females. This score indicated that the females in this group were more likely to be abusing alcohol or drugs. This result suggested that although this group of patients were likely to be affected by substance or alcohol misuse problems, females were more likely to have misused drugs and/or alcohol than were the males.

The mean score for criminality was above the average for controls and within the average for prisoners. This was a group of individuals who were more than likely to be involved in offending or criminal behaviour as part of their general behaviours. When the mean score for males was separated from the mean score for females, it showed that the females were far more inclined to be criminally minded than were the males. These results suggested that this was a high risk group of individuals who were more than likely to have had an index offence and who were more likely to continue such patterns of behaviour, as part of their normal general everyday activity. This was a group of people who would re-offend and remain a danger or high risk to themselves or others.

The mean score on the Lie scale was within the average range for 'normals', males and females. This suggested that these results could, in clinical terms, be considered as reliable, reasonable and acceptable responses from this patient group.

The differences in mean scores for 16 personality factors at the first assessment (Time 1) as compared with mean scores at the six month assessment (Time 2) are shown in Table 6.4.

The group's performance on the eight factors showed that the individuals in this group were generally detached from the wider society. They were less stable emotionally, changeable and easily affected by feelings. These were individuals who tend to be highly aggressive, stubborn and would use violence and aggression as a means to control or dominate their world. This was a group who were fully aware of what they were doing yet failed to respect tra-

Table 6.4 Findings from 16 Personality Factors overtime

Factor	Time 1 mean scores N=13	Time 2 mean scores N=6
A	4.62	4.83
B	4.38	5.00
C	3.08	3.33
E	6.08	6.17
F	5.23	4.17
G	5.85	4.33
H	5.85	5.50
I	5.23	4.33
L	6.23	6.83
M	5.77	5.17
N	6.54	5.50
O	6.31	6.17
Q1	5.62	6.67
Q2	7.46	7.50
Q3	4.38	4.33
Q4	6.38	6.83

ditional views or consider alternative ways of dealing with their problems other than by violence or aggression. They would not hesitate to attack people or damage property in order to achieve objectives associated with the main or secondary characteristics of their complex behaviour profile. They tend to abide by their own rules and do not volunteer compliance. The difference in mean scores for the eight factors in this test at Time 1 and Time 2 was small (0.16) and fell within the normal range of standard deviation. These underlying psychological and behavioural factors remained stable over time in this group though some social behaviours changed. These findings suggest that these individuals might comply, if guided or influenced to do so, by clear and identifiable boundaries. However, once the boundaries are removed it is likely that the main and subordinate characteristics of their complex behaviour profile will re-emerge again and again.

Social and behavioural factors

Attention was given to the CSU's aim to help this group of individuals to achieve an optimal level of social functioning. Assessment of their level of disability was derived from the set rating scales in HoNOS, LUNSERS and the Lancaster Quality of Life which assisted in the development of individual care plans. The total findings suggest that this was a group that showed a high level of detachment from social norms and acceptable behaviours. This was a group with distorted views and atypical social behaviours which formed part of their complex behaviour profile. The indication was that this was a group of individuals with very profound needs. Targets were set for each individual to achieve within the CSU's therapeutic community and these were measured and evaluated in terms of indicators of change in their social behaviour over time. The global findings are shown in Fig. 6.2. These showed that over 73% of targets were achieved by individuals in this group. There were signs of less detachment, distortion and atypical social behaviours. This result suggested that the observable changes in patients' behaviour were associated

Percentage of targets achieved/not achieved for all patients (*N*=13)

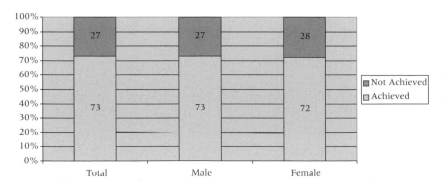

Fig. 6.2 Targets achieved

with *state* personality factors only; but maladaptive behaviours that were associated with underlying personality *traits* factors remained unchanged.

Summary

In summary, a psychological research model was employed in the investigation of a small group of individuals who formed part of a much larger longitudinal study of patients with complex behaviour who were admitted to a CSU for help. The initial investigation identified the complex behaviour profile which showed that individuals had a varied mixture of comorbidity that attracted the label dual diagnosis from a medical model perspective. The psychological research model however, established that other aspects of the patients' behaviour could not be excluded from the profile as these shared equal status in the world of individuals who have very profound needs.

Psychological testing detected certain cognitive and behavioural factors in this group. This confirmed the hypothesis that certain psychological and behavioural factors do exist in patients with complex behaviour who are labelled 'dual diagnosis'. When various tests were repeated over time, the mean scores suggest confirmation of the second hypothesis—that detected psychological and behavioural factors act as determinants of the complex behaviour profile. The scores derived from some individual test scores confirmed the results of other psychological tests used in the battery, both on detection of factors and on the observed difference(s) among females and males in the said psychological factors and likely accompanying behavioural factors in this population.

Apart from the different attributes and variables highlighted from differences in the specific test scores, the overall results suggest that females were a more hostile unstable group than males. They were far more skilled at disguising their maladaptive behaviours than were the males; and, to a large extent far more dangerous in terms of their history of offending behaviours. Yet, the males in this group, who were generally of low ability, were more likely to be seen by others as presenting a greater danger, more aggression and more violence than the females. It would seem that gender stereotyping may lead to faulty perception of male vs. female related complex behaviour. If not acknowledged, this could, in some cases, affect clinical judgement, and present a difficulty in risk assessment, risk management and risk harnessment. Raters may underrate women's potential for violence and dangerousness.

It was also hypothesised that detected psychological and behavioural characteristics of the complex behaviour profile of patients who are admitted to a therapeutic community setting will change over time. However, although patients achieved over 73% of targets in terms of their social functioning, the findings from the test and re-test data from various measures could not fully confirm this hypothesis. The 16PF findings over time suggested that identified behavioural changes in patients may be associated with state personality factors only. These results suggest that the detected psychological and behavioural factors can not be excluded from the assessment of individuals who are dually diagnosed since these factors may play an important part in determining the resistant nature of the patients' enduring mental illness, criminal or offending behaviour, maladaptive behaviour and poor level of social functioning. The underlying factors that may have been responsible for the individual's need to be in a secure environment would not necessarily change over time. In short, the main and subordinate characteristics of the complex behaviour profile incorporating the offending behaviours of both males and females would remain unchanged, though dormant, in the person so affected; and, given the appropriate integration of circumstances, the offending behaviour could repeatedly manifest itself as a continuing danger and risk to the individual and to the public.

Discussion

There are many different models for complex behaviours (e.g. Eysenck 1960a; Siegler & Osmond 1966; Siegler *et al.* 1969). It is universally known that psychiatrists do not consistently apply a specific model and many move from one model to another between diagnosis and treatment without realising they have done so (McGuire 1973). This practice has continued despite some earlier attempts at more objective ways of forming clinical judgements (Moore 1929; Lubin 1950; Rao 1952, 1962; Meehl 1954, 1965; Eysenck 1955; Greenhouse 1965; Lyerly 1965; Rome *et al.* 1965; Torgerson 1965; Nathan 1967; Spitzer & Endicott 1968; Hope 1969; Pilowsky *et al.* 1969).

These inconsistencies in psychiatry highlight the difficulties surrounding attaching a dual diagnosis label to complex behaviour. However, there is a continuing tendency to rely on nosological models as the basis for conceptualising and representing psychiatric-type phenomena. The ICD-10 model (WHO 1992) describes the phenomenon as a descriptive class of disorders. This approach has also led to some confusion in the way puzzling pathology, or complex behaviour, have been perceived. In some instances more than ten different diagnostic labels were generated to describe the unusual presentation of a group of patients (Stone 1980; Chaham 1985). Goldstein (1983), among others (e.g. Wheeler & Walton 1987; Kroll 1988; Herman *et al.* 1989), drew attention to the need for clinicians to attend to the multiple external and internal stresses, other than medical, that the individual brings to the situation. In addition, it is also desirable for clinicians, service providers and lay persons alike to be cognisant of the notion of 'dual-diagnosis-amplification' and its implications.

It is observed that some earlier writers, such as Kernberg (1967, 1975, 1984), did not view presenting problems, or overt symptoms and traits, as reliable indicators of borderline psychiatric conditions. This acknowledgement, in the writer's opinion, reinforces the view that the label 'dual diagnosis' may serve to minimise or distract from a full consideration of the individual's overall complex behaviour profile and lead to a reduction of emphasis on individual needs. The result might be a perpetuation of the idea of 'needs as complex' rather than a promotion of the more important premise of 'needs as profound'.

Comas-Dias and Minrath (1985) commented on the strains of biculturalism that may create or reinforce split images of the self, loss of centrality, confusion, fear of dissolution, and identity diffusion. Chestang (1972) described the depressive effects of imposed devaluation on the individual and Lewis (1984) described the self-alienation effects of externally inflicted negative labelling on lesbian women. Goldstein (1990) suggests that the development of symptoms such as depression, substance abuse and suicidal behaviour may be a consequence of efforts to cope with identity conflicts that stem from conflicts between the individual and society. The existence of more than one of these features in the same person is therefore deserving of a greater understanding of their complex behaviour profile.

As the findings in the study here showed, complex behaviour is multifaceted. Each facet can be ambiguous and reflective of a positive or negative self. Many early theorists have remarked on this uniqueness in the individual (e.g. Freud's (1922) notion of the conscious and the unconscious). Stern (1938) introduced the term 'borderline personality' to describe patients who manifested mixed pathology. Deutsch (1942) coined the term 'as if' personality to describe the phenomenon. Schmideberg (1947) suggested that the characterised instability in the person was a stable form of personality disorder. Nine features of the phenomenon were highlighted: an inability to tolerate routine and regularity; a tendency to break many of the rules of social convention; lateness for appointments; inability to associate freely; poor motivation for treatment; failure to develop meaningful insight; chaotic lives; criminal acts and difficulty in establishing emotional contact. Frosch (1960) referred to those who shared certain characteristics as having a 'psychotic character'. There has also been a recognition that patients can move between conditions (Knight 1953). Grinker *et al.* (1968) identified four main characteristics of patients who were difficult to diagnose: anger, defeat in affectionate/interpersonal relationships, absence of consistent self-identity; and depression. The case strengthens for attention to be focused on identifying complex behaviour in terms of its main and subordinate characteristics.

The findings from the present study are reflected in some of this early work which drew attention to the multifaceted and functional nature of complex behaviour. The search is for more clarity of the way that the individual behaves. The indication is that the behaviour is complex behaviour with main and subordinate characteristics and with two or more problems/illnesses/disorders so labelled in terms of dual diagnosis (e.g. schizophrenic–alcoholic? or alcoholic–schizophrenic?). Rapaport *et al.* (1945–46) remind us that patients' performance on psychometric tests may resemble neurotic patients on some of the tests and schizophrenic patients on others. Thus, who, and what subjective criteria, decide the order of the labels is problematic.

There is a strong case for the use of a psychological research model to explore the uniqueness of the individual's complex behaviour profile. An individual's risk does not remain constant. The application of the psychological research model provides some answers which may help determine the level of dangerousness posed by these individuals and how it might be managed and/or harnessed, as well as how their profound needs might be met and their future behaviour determined. The findings suggest that individuals with complex behaviour profiles sometimes express opposing needs (e.g. ambivalence) with related features (e.g. aggression, violence, dangerousness) deserving of psychological understanding, intervention and facilitation of change. A risk assessment should not be seen as a 'be all and end all' nor should the imposition of risk management strategies. While acknowledging the problem of identifying false positives, clinicians should be made aware of factors in an individual's complex behaviour profile that might be associated with the harnessing of behaviour. Thus, apart from medical model activity associated with the label dual diagnosis and the recognition of the influence of historical and demographic variables, regular patient reviews should take account of the recent or current status of psychological and behavioural factors associated with the individual's complex behaviour profile.

The data from other measures (HoNOS, Lancashire Quality of Life, Lunsers, etc.) highlighted serious deficits in the social functioning of these patients. The females were found to be more greatly affected by behavioural problems than were the males in most areas. The results from the Lunsers also showed that they required higher levels of medication than did the males in order to achieve the same effect or to maintain a similar level of stability within the therapeutic setting and achieve more satisfaction with their quality of life, as fixed within the framework of boundaries. Rapoport (1960) described four features of life in the therapeutic community that he felt were of importance in the facilitation of change: permissiveness, communality, democracy and reality confrontation. As reflected in the literature, there seems to be little doubt that certain issues do arise in therapeutic communities. It was noted that not all therapeutic communities are the same (De Leon 1995). There is a sense of uniqueness around each therapeutic community which needs to be understood (Rapoport 1960; Bloor & McKegancy 1987). This group of patients was exposed to the rehabilitatory/ socio-dynamic approach within the therapeutic community where the staff represented different facets of the community life. They integrated at a less detached level and showed their own feelings, as appropriate. There was more emphasis on confrontation of the patient about their behaviour, here and now, than on interpretation. The patient was an active agent in treatment (Jones 1959, 1962a,b).

An assessment of the achievement of goals, as a measure of change in patients' maladaptive behaviour, showed that these patients achieved 73% of set targets. These results suggested that the uniqueness of the CSU therapeutic community approach was effective in facilitating change in some social aspects of their behaviour. This finding is in keeping with those of Hipwell *et al.* (2000) who found that substance misusers with mental health problems used day services to acquire help with social difficulties but their mental health problem remained unchallenged. The patients' subjective accounts confirmed that certain aspects of the therapeutic programme helped change some of their detached and atypical social behaviours. The strength and power of the community principle stabilised the main and subordinate characteristics of their complex behaviour and effected changes in their social behaviour. The ongoing reality of risk and the tendency towards repeated acts of dangerousness associated with this patient group should be acknowledged. There is justification for the public to be concerned, just as clinicians ought to be, because the factors associated with the main and subordinate characteristics of any individual's complex behaviour profile remain unchanged. The aim now ought to be for clinicians to gain a greater understanding of the complex behaviour profile of patients and to avoid any likely misperception of the phenomenon in exchange for a medically determined dual diagnosis label.

Conclusion

It was acknowledged in the foregoing that the findings presented in this chapter related to a small portion of the overall data from a much larger longitudinal study. However, the reported results so far questioned the usefulness of ascribing the label 'dual diagnosis' to patients with complex behaviour. The study detected certain underlying psychological and behavioural factors, associated with the main or subordinate characteristics of complex behaviour, present in patients who were labelled dual diagnosis. These factors remained stable over time. This finding indicated that patients with complex behaviour profiles are likely to show no fundamental change in either the main or subordinate characteristics of their complex behaviour over time despite achieving some stability in their social behaviour in the short or medium term. These individuals are therefore likely to remain dangerous and a risk to themselves and to the public once removed from an environment where boundaries are in force. The retention of potential dangerousness in the individual affected can not be minimised. These results suggest that more encouragement should be given to the use of a psychological research model in an attempt at understanding and dealing with the influence of certain psychological and behavioural factors upon the main or subordinate characteristic of complex behaviour.

This is a strong call for the application of a psychological model because despite attempts to achieve diagnostic symmetry between psychiatrists (ICD-10, WHO 1992; DSM-1 V, APA 1994) there is still a tendency for clinical judgements to be culture-bound and person-perceptive in nature. Attempts at a shared understanding of the label dual diagnosis, in terms of comorbidity, remains problematic. To differentiate complex behaviour purely in terms of its psychiatric concomitants may be a fruitless exercise. It is likely that a psychological research model would enable a study of the subtler components of psychological and behavioural factors associated with complex behaviour to be achieved. It will highlight the intra- and inter-underlying psychological and behavioural factors present in the individual and any detectable differences in an apparent comorbidity. The desire on the part of some clinicians to persist in the labelling of patients as 'dual diagnosis', may be too hasty. It is my contention that the ascription of a mixture of questionable psychiatric labels to the subject as being dual diagnosis would not be able to achieve the same outcome as would the application of a psychological research model.

The current debate should take account of the value of the psychological research model in detecting psychological and behavioural factors in individuals which underly their manifested complex behaviour. This model suggests that the complexity of the presenting behaviour should be examined, assessed and evaluated in any attempt at assessing and meeting the individual's profound needs. This is not necessarily achieved through a medical model. A number of publications (e.g. Caudill 1952; Belknap 1956; Goffman 1961) strongly challenged the medical model in this respect by emphasising the role of the social structure of units, the influence of the social system of institutions and patient culture in the outcome of care of patients in a psychiatric setting.

Paul and Lentz (1977) posited the notion of the principle of expectancy, i.e. the belief that the social and physical environment for patients who require some degree of security will have an effect on their subsequent behaviour, relationship and aspirations. The challenge of testing this hypothesis was reflected in the work of Weaver *et al.* (1978a, b) who reported that a number of patients' disruptive behaviours on a locked ward were a function, in part, of a set of expectations, beliefs and attitudes held by nurses about the patients they were nursing and that the type of behaviours demonstrated by patients were associated with nurses' beliefs that the mentally ill are not responsible for their behaviour, that there is little hope for improvement and that people who are admitted to a unit for the disturbed are going to act in a disturbed manner. The focus should now be widened and the concept of 'disturbed behaviour' clarified. The findings of the present investigation suggest that it may not be the carer's expectation that is responsible for the maintenance of disturbed behaviour. The results from repeated measures suggest that the disturbed behaviour is present within the framework of the main and subordinate characteristics of the individual's complex behaviour and not necessarily determined by a carer's expectations. There is also the matter that some variables within the profile are unlikely to change over time irrespective of the intervention or the carer's beliefs. The results from analysis of the 16 PF and other data over time indicated that there were no significant changes in certain underlying psychological and behavioural factors. It would seem from these results that the observed changes in patient behaviour were associated with social behaviours which were linked to STAI-T factors only. This idea of expectancy and disturbed behaviour, as highlighted by Paul and Lentz (1977) therefore appears to relate to the social aspects of behaviour.

The findings of the present study suggest that although some elements of an individual's complex behaviour profile are likely to remain stable within a setting of boundaries, aspects of the main or subordinate characteristics of their behaviour will re-emerge, at any given time. The indication is that patients with complex behaviour who require admission to a secure setting are likely to remain dangerous and retain a high risk of repeating the offending maladaptive behaviours once the boundaries are removed. Such behaviours, it would seem from the findings, generally remain unchanged though stable and dormant during a period of therapeutic or custodial intervention.

Patients with complex behaviour form a relatively dangerous high risk group of individuals with many problems. Actual responses to treatment, or behavioural reactions, can not necessarily be predicted. The findings from the present study have drawn attention to the importance of identifying the main and subordinate characteristics of the complex behaviour and the associated psychological and behavioural factors of the individual referred. There ought not to be a sole reliance on the psychiatric label ascribed to the referred individual, as a 'dual diagnosis'.

Any combination of psychiatric labels may be found in a forensic setting. The present findings suggest that the usefulness of a dual diagnosis label attached to this category of patient is yet to be determined. What seems to be of more value is the application of a psychological research model to establish the complex behaviour profile. The profiles which were derived for this cohort of patients suggest that the underlying psychological and behavioural factors of patients with dual diagnosis labels should be taken seriously in any attempt at examining the influence of these factors on effecting change in the main and subordinate characteristics of their complex behaviour. It thus becomes more important for all interested parties to be more aware of the psychological and behavioural factors of the person and what he or she is likely to do than of what labels psychiatrists choose to describe them.

Key points

There is a need for an expansion of the debate on the complexity of behaviour and associated profoundness of needs.

• Questioning of perceptions of 'dual diagnosis' needs to continue and the usefulness of the recent assertions about its clinical applicability need to be contested.

• Systematic exploration of the components of complex behaviour need to be undertaken in different settings and across different time periods of an individual's history.

• The notion of 'dual-diagnosis-amplification' is posited. There is a need for clinicians, service providers and lay persons alike to acknowledge and take responsibility for its implications.

• The complex behaviour profile defines the likely process of service provision and construction in accordance with the individual presentation of self.

• The psychological research model presents an opportunity to explore the concept of complex behaviour in terms of addressing issues beyond risk assessment and risk management. It draws attention to the need for a new direction and focus on risk harnessment, i.e. the harnessing of the ongoing reality of risk; and encourages renewed interests in finding more answers to questions about dangerousness.

References

American Psychiatric Association (1994) *Diagnostic and Statistical Manual of Mental Disorders*, 4th edn. American Psychiatric Association, Washington DC.

Ash, P. (1949) The reliability of psychiatric diagnosis. *Journal of Abnormal and Social Psychology* **44**, 272–276.

Barker, C., Pistrang, N. & Elliott, R. (1995) *Research Methods in Clinical and Counselling Psychology*. Wiley, Chichester.

Beck, A.T. (1962) Reliability of psychiatric diagnoses: 1. A critique of systematic studies. *American Journal of Psychiatry* **119**, 210–216.

Beck, A.T., Epstein, N., Brown, G. & Steer, R.A. (1988) An inventory for measuring clinical anxiety: Psychometric properties. *Journal of Consulting and Clinical Psychology* **56**, 893–897.

Beck, A.T., Rush, A.J., Shaw, B.F. & Emery, G. (1979) *Cognitive Therapy of Depression*. Guilford Press, New York.

Belknap, I. (1956) *Human Problems of a State Mental Hospital*. McGraw-Hill, New York.

Bell, M.D. & Ryan, E.R. (1985) Where can therapeutic community ideals be realised? An examination of three treatment environments. *Hospital and Community Psychiatry* **36**, 12.

Bloor, M.J. & McKeganacy, N.P. (1987) Outstanding practices: Evaluative aspects of a descriptive sociological study of eight contrasting therapeutic communities. *International Journal of Therapeutic Communities* **8**, 4.

Caine, T.M., Foulds, G.A. & Hope, K. (1967) *Manual of the Hostility and Direction of Hostility Questionnaire (HDHQ)*. University of London Press, London.

Carpenter, L. & Brockington, I.F. (1980) A study of mental illness in Asians, West Indians and Africans living in Manchester. *British Journal of Psychiatry* **137**, 201–205.

Caudill, W. (1952) Social structure and interaction processes on a psychiatric ward. *American Journal of Orthopsychiatry* **22**, 314–334.

Chaham, P. (1985) *Treatment of Borderline Personality*. Jason Aronson, New York.

Chestang, L. (1972) Character development in a hostile environment. In: M.Bloom (ed.) (1980) *Life Span Development: Bases for Preventive and Interventive Helping*. Macmillan, New York, pp. 40–50.

Clark, D.H. (1965) The therapeutic community—concept, practice and future. *British Journal of Psychiatry* **111**, 947–954.

Cochrane, R. (1977) Immigration and mental hospital admission. *Social Psychiatry* **12**, 25–35.

Comas-Dias, L. & Minrath, M. (1985) Psychotherapy with ethnic borderline clients. *Psychotherapy* **22**, 418–426.

Day, J., Wood, G., Dewey, M. & Bentall, R. (1995) A self-rating scale for measuring neuroleptic side-effects. *British Journal of Psychiatry* **166**, 650–653.

De Leon, G. (1995) Residential therapeutic communities in the mainstream: diversity and issues. *Journal of Psychoactive Drugs* **27** (1), 3–15.

Department of Health (1992) *Health of the Nation Rating Scales*. HMSO, London.

Department of Health Social Security (1983) *Mental Health Act*. HMSO, London.

Deutsch, H. (1942) Some forms of emotional disturbance and their relationship to schizophrenia. *Psychoanalytic Quarterly* **11**, 301–321.

Drake, R.E. & Wallach, M.A. (1989) Substance abuse among the chronic mentally ill. *Hospital and Community Psychiatry* **40**, 1041–1046.

Eysenck, H.J. (1955) Psychiatric diagnosis as a psychological and statistical problem. *Psychological Report* **1**, 3–17.

Eysenck, H.J. (1960) Classification and the problem of diagnosis. In: H.J. Eysenck (ed.) *The Handbook of Abnormal Psychology*. Pitman Medical, London.

Eysenck, H.J. & Eysenck, S.B.G. (1975) *Eysenck Personality Questionnaire—Revised*. University of London Press, London.

Filstead, W.J. & Rossi, J.J. (1973) *The Therapeutic Community*. Behavioural Publications, New York.

Freud, S. (1922) *Group Psychology and the Analysis of the Ego*. International Psychoanalytic Press, London.

Frosch, J. (1960) Psychotic character. *Journal of the American Psychoanalytic Association* **8**, 554–551.

Genders, E. & Player, E. (1995) *Grendon: A study of a therapeutic prison*. Oxford University Press, Oxford.

Goffman, E. (1961) *Asylums: Essays on the Social Situation of Mental Patients and Other Inmates*. Doubleday, New York.

Goffman, E. (1968) *Asylums*. Penguin Books, Harmondsworth.

Goldberg, D. (1978) *Manual of the General Health Questionnaire*. NFER-NELSON Publishing Co., Windsor.

Goldstein, E.G. (1983) Clinical and ecological approaches to the borderline client. *Social Casework—the Journal of Contemporary Social Work* **64**, 353–362.

Goldstein, E.G. (1990) Borderline disorders. *Clinical Models and Techniques*. Guilford Press, New York.

Good, D.A. & Watts, F.N. (1989) Qualitative research. In: G. Parry & F.N. Watts (eds) *Behavioural and Mental Health Research: a Handbook of Skill and Methods*. Lawrence Erlbaum Associates, Hove.

Greenhouse, S.W. (1965) On the meaning of discrimination, classification, mixture and clustering in statistics. In: M.M. Katz, J.O. Cole & W.E. Barton (eds) *The Role and Methodology of Classification in Psychiatry and Psychopathology*. US Department of Health, Education and Welfare, Chevy Chase, Md.

Grinker, R.R., Werble, B. & Drye, R. (1968) *The Borderline Syndrome*. Basic Books, New York.

Gunderson, J.G. (1983) An overview of modern milieu therapy. In: J.G. Gunderson, O.A. Will & L.R. Mosher (eds) *Principles and Practices of Milieu Therapy*. Aronson, New York.

Harrison, G., Incichen, B., Smith, J. & Morgan, H.G. (1984) Psychiatric hospital admissions in Bristol, 11, Social and clinical aspects of compulsory admission. *British Journal of Psychiatry* **145**, 605–611.

Harrison, G., Owens, D., Holton, A., Neilson, D. & Boot, D. (1988) A perspective study of severe mental disorder in Afro-Caribbean patients. *Psychological Medicine* **18**, 643–657.

Herman, J.L., Perry, J.C. & van der Kolk, B. (1989) Childhood trauma in borderline personality disorder. *American Journal of Psychiatry* **146**, 490–495.

Hipwell, A.E., Singh, K. & Clark, A. (2000) Substance misuse among clients with severe and enduring mental illness: service utilization and implications for clinical management. *Journal of Mental Health* **9** (1), 37–50.

Home Office (1975) *Report of the Committee on Mentally Disordered Offenders (Butler Report) (Cmnd 6244)*. HMSO, London.

Hope, K. (1969) The complete analysis of a data matrix. *British Journal of Psychiatry* **115**, 1069–1079.

Horsley, J.A. (1982) *Mutual Goal Setting in Patient Care: Conduct and utilization of research in nursing*. Harcourt Brace Jovanovich, New York.

Hunt, W.A., Wittson, C.L. & Hunt, E.B.A. (1953) Theoretical and practical analysis of the diagnostic process. In: P.J. Hoch & J. Zubin (eds) *Current Problems in Psychiatric Diagnosis*. Grune and Stratton, New York.

Institute of Personality and Ability Testing (1972) *16 Personality Factor Questionnaire (16PF)*. IPAT, Champaign, Ill.

Jones, M. (1959) Toward a clarification of the therapeutic community concept. *British Journal of Medical Psychology* **32**, 200–205.

Jones, M. (1962a) *Social Psychiatry in the Community*. Charles Thomas, Springfield.

Jones, M. (1962b) Training in social psychiatry at the ward level. *American Journal of Psychiatry* **118**, 705–708.

Keppel, G. (1991) *Design and Analysis: A research handbook*, 3rd edn. Prentice Hall, Englewood Cliffs, NJ.

Kernberg, O.F. (1967) Borderline personality organization. *Journal of the American Psychoanalytic Association* **15**, 641–685.

Kernberg, O.F. (1975) *Borderline Conditions and Pathological Narcissism*. Jason Aronson, New York.

Kernberg, O.F. (1984) *Severe Personality Disorders*. Yale University Press, New Haven.

Kiev, A. (1965) Psychiatric morbidity of West Indian immigrants in an urban group practice. *British Journal of Psychiatry* **111**, 51–56.

Kirk, R.E. (1982) *Experimental Design: Procedures for the behavioural sciences*, 2nd edn. Brooks/Cole, Belmont, CA.

Knight, R.P. (1953) Borderline states. *Bulletin of the Menninger Clinic* **17**, 1–12.

Knowles, J. (1995) Therapeutic communities in today's world. *Therapeutic Communities: the International Journal for Therapeutic and Supportive Organizations* **16** (2), 97–102.

Kraepelin, E. (1909–13) *Psychiatry*, 8th edn. Thieme, Leipzig.

Kreitman, N. (1961) The reliability of psychiatric diagnosis. *Journal of Mental Science* **107**, 876–886.

Kreitman, N., Sainsbury, P., Morrissey, J., Towers, J. & Scrivener, J. (1961) The reliability of psychiatric assessment: an analysis. *Journal of Mental Science* **107**, 887–908.

Kroll, J. (1988) *The Challenge of the Borderline Personality*. Norton, New York.

Lewis, L.A. (1984) The coming out process of lesbians: Integrating a stable identity. *Social Work* **29**, 464–469.

Littlewood, R. (1988) Towards an inter-cultural therapy: some preliminary observations. *Journal of Social Work Practice* **Nov**, 8–19.

Littlewood, R. & Lipsedge, M. (1981) Psychiatric illness amongst British Afro-Caribbeans. *British Medical Journal* **296** (950), 951.

London, M. (1986) Mental illness amongst immigrant minorities in the United Kingdom. *British Journal of Psychiatry* **149**, 265–273.

Lubin, A. (1950) Some contributions to the testing of psychological hypotheses by means of statistical multivariate analysis. Unpubl. PhD Thesis, University of London.

Lyerly, S.B. (1965) A survey of some empirical clustering procedures. In: M.M. Katz, J.O. Cole & W.E. Barton (eds) *The Role and Methodology of Classification in Psychiatry and Psychopathology*. US Department of Health, Education and Welfare, Chevy Chase, Md.

Main, T.F. (1946) The hospital as a therapeutic community. *Bulletin of the Menninger Clinic* **10**, 66–70.

Main, T.F. (1967) Knowledge, learning and freedom from thought. *Australian N Zeitscrift für Journal of Psychiatry* **1**, 64–71.

Main, T.F. (1983) The concept of the therapeutic community: variations and vicissitudes. In: M. Pines (ed.) *The Evolution of Group Analysis*. Routledge and Kegan Paul Ltd, London.

Maxwell, A. (1973) Psychiatric illness: some inferences from symptomatology. *British Journal of Psychiatry* **122**, 252–258.

McGovern, D. & Cope, R. (1987) The compulsory detention of males of different ethnic groups with reference to offender patients. *British Journal of Psychiatry* **150**, 505–512.

McGuire, R.J. (1973) Classification and the problem of diagnosis. In: H.J. Eysenck (ed.) *Handbook of Abnormal Psychology*. Pitman Medical, London.

Meehl, P.E. (1954) *Clinical versus Statistical Prediction*. University of Minnesota Press, Minneapolis.

Meehl, P.E. (1965) Seer over sign: the first good example. *Journal of Experimental Research* **1**, 27–32.

Moore, T.V. (1929) The empirical determination of certain syndromes underlying praecox and manic depressive psychoses. *American Journal of Psychiatry* **9**, 719–738.

Nathan, P.E. (1967) *Cues, Decisions and Diagnosis*. Academic Press, New York.

Parry, G. (1992) Improving psychotherapy services: Applications of research, audit and evaluation. *British Journal of Clinical Psychology* **31**, 3–19.

Parsons, T. (1937) *The Structure of Social Action*. McGraw-Hill, New York.

Parsons, T. (1951) *The Social System*. Free Press, New York.

Parsons, T. (1995) The sick role and the role of physicians reconsidered. *Health Society* **53**, 257–258.

Paul, G.L. & Lentz, R.J. (1977) *Psychosocial Treatment of Chronic Mental Patients. Milieu Vs Social Learning Programs*. Harvard University Press, Cambridge, MA.

Perkins, R.E. (1994) *Merton Rehabilitation Team Multidisciplinary Clinical Audit Project*. Pathfinder Mental Health Services NHS Trust, London.

Perkins, R.E. & Russell, L. (1988) *The Wandsworth and Merton Long Term Care Assessment*. Pathfinder Community and Specialist Mental Health Services, London.

Pilowsky, I., Levine, S. & Boulton, D.M. (1969) The classification of depression by numerical taxonomy. *British Journal of Psychiatry* **115**, 937–945.

Pinsent, J. (1963) Morbidity in an immigrant population. *The Lancet* **1**, 437–438.

Preston, C.A. & Vinev, L.L. (1984) Self- and ideal-self-perception of drug addicts in therapeutic communities. *International Journal of Addiction* **19**, 805–818.

Rao, C.R. (1952) *Advanced Statistical Methods in Biometric Research*. John Wiley & Sons, New York.

Rao, C.R. (1962) Use of discriminant and allied functions in multivariate analysis. *Sankhya* **22**, 317–338.

Rapaport, D., Gill, M.M. & Schafer, R. (1945–46) *Diagnostic Psychological Testing* (2 Volumes). Year Book Publishers, Chicago.

Rapoport, R. (1960) *Community as Doctor*. Tavistock, London.

Roach, F. (1992) Community mental health services for black and ethnic minorities. *Counselling Psychology Quarterly* **5** (3), 277–290.

Rome, H.P., Mataya, P., Pearson, J.S., Swenson, W.M. & Brannick, T.L. (1965) Automatic personality assessment. In: R.W. Stacy & B.D. Waxman (eds) *Computers in Biomedical Research*. Academic Press, New York.

Rotter, J.B. (1966) Generalized expectancies for internal versus external control of reinforcement. *Psychological Monographs* **80** (1), 1–28.

Rotter, J.B. (1971) External control and internal control. *Psychology Today* **5** (1) (37–42), 58–59.

Russell, W.M. (1945) *The New York Hospital: A history of the psychiatric service, 1771–1936*. Columbia University Press, New York.

Russell, J., ed. (1993) *Alcohol and Crime*. Mental Health Foundation, London.

Sandifer, M.G., Pettus, C. & Quade, D. (1964) A study of psychiatric diagnosis. *Journal of Nervous and Mental Disease* **139**, 350–356.

Santana, S., Fisher, N. & Perkins, R.E. (1997) *Evaluating Outcome in a Rehabilitation and Continuing Care Service for People with Serious and Enduring Mental Health Problems*. Pathfinder Community and Specialist Mental Health Services, London.

Schimmel, P. (1997) Swimming against the tide? A review of the therapeutic community. *Australian and New Zealand Journal of Psychiatry* **31** (1), 120–127.

Schmideberg, M. (1947) The treatment of psychopaths and borderline patients. *American Journal of Psychotherapy* **1**, 45–55.

Schmidt, H.O. & Fonda, C.P. (1956) The reliability of psychiatric diagnosis: a new look. *Journal of Abnormal and Social Psychology* **52**, 262–267.

Siegler, M. & Osmond, H. (1966) Models of madness. *British Journal of Psychiatry* **112**, 1193–1203.

Siegler, M., Osmond, H. & Mann, H. (1969) Lang's models of madness. *British Journal of Psychiatry* **115**, 947–958.

Spielberger, C.D. (1968) *Self-Evaluation Questionnaire*. Consulting Psychologists Press, Inc., Palo Alto, CA.

Spitzer, R.L. & Endicott, J. (1968) DIAGNO: a computer program for psychiatric diagnosis utilising the differential diagnostic procedure. *Archives of General Psychiatry* **18**, 746–756.

Stanton, A.H. & Schwartz, M.S. (1954) *The Mental Hospital*. Basic Books, New York.

Stern, A. (1938) Psychoanalytic investigation of and therapy in a borderline group of neuroses. *Psychoanalytic Quarterly* **7**, 467–489.

Stone, M.H. (1980) *The Borderline Syndrome*. McGraw-Hill, New York.

Stubblebin, J.M. (1973) The therapeutic community—a further formulation. In: J.J. Rossi & W.J. Filstead (eds) *The Therapeutic Community—A Source Book of Readings*. Behavioural Publications, New York.

Taylor, S.J. & Bosdan, R. (1984) *Introduction to Qualitative Research Methods. The Search for Meanings*, 2nd edn. Wiley, New York.

Taylor, S.M., Galanter, M., Dermatis, H., Spivack, N. & Egelko, S. (1997) Dual diagnosis patients in the modified therapeutic community: Does a criminal history hinder adjustment or treatment? *Journal of Addictive Diseases* **16** (3), 31–38.

Torgerson, W.S. (1965) Multidimensional representation of similarity structures. In: M.M. Katz, J.O. Cole & W.E. Barton (eds) *The Role and Methodology of Classification in Psychiatry and Psychopathology*. US Department of Health, Education & Welfare, Chevy Chase, Md.

Trauser, T. (1984) The current status of the therapeutic community. *British Journal of Medical Psychology* **57**, 71–79.

Ward, C.H., Beck, A.T., Mendelson, M., Mock, J.E. & Erbaugh, J.K. (1962) The psychiatric nomenclature: reasons for diagnostic disagreement. *Archives of General Psychiatry* **7**, 198–205.

Weaver, S.M., Armstrong, N.E., Broome, A.K. & Stewart, L. (1978a) Behavioural principle applied to a security ward. *Nursing Times* **5**, 22–24.

Weaver, S.M., Broome, A.K. & Kat, B.J.B. (1978b) Some patterns of disturbed behaviour in a closed ward environment. *Journal of Advanced Nursing* **3**, 251–263.

Wechler, D. (1981) *Wechsler Adult Intelligence Scale—Revised. The Psychological Corporation*. Harcourt Brace Jovanovich, New York.

Westreich, L., Galanter, M., Lifshutz, H., Metzger, E.J. & Silberstein, C. (1996) A modified therapeutic community for the dually diagnosed—Greenhouse Program at Bellevue Hospital. *Journal of Substance Abuse Treatment* **13** (60), 533–536.

Wheeler, B.K. & Walton, E. (1987) Personality disturbances of adult incest victims. *Social Casework: the Journal of Contempory Social Work* **68**, 597–602.

Whiteley, J.S. (1986) Sociotherapy and psychotherapy in the treatment of personality disorder. *Journal of the Royal Society of Medicine* 79, December.

Wilkins, L.A. (1969) Social deviance: social policy. *Action and Research*. Tavistock, London.

Wilmer, H. (1958) *Social Psychiatry in Action: A Therapeutic Community*. Springfield.

World Health Organisation (1953) *Therapeutic Communities*. WHO, Geneva.

Zublin, J. (1967) Classification of the behaviour disorders. *Annual Review of Psychology* **18**.

Part 2: Context and Practice

7: The Challenge of Shared Care

Mike Flanagan

Introduction

Despite more than a decade of research, there continues to be a poor response to the needs of those with comorbid substance misuse and mental illness by drug treatment agencies and general psychiatric services. The Royal College of Psychiatrists has acknowledged this concern, and called for integrated treatment systems for those with comorbid problems (Royal College of Psychiatrists 2000). Leading research into models of service delivery for this group has most commonly been carried out in the United States. The emphasis has been on the development of integrated treatment where mental illness and substance misuse are treated simultaneously by the same clinician from a single, ultra-specialist dual diagnosis team (Drake *et al.* 1998; Mueser *et al.* 1998; George & Krystal 2000). However, a recent review of randomised trials of integrated programmes for mental illness and substance use problems concluded the current momentum for integrated treatment systems is not based on good evidence, and that no one programme is superior to another (Ley *et al.* 2000).

In many respects, substance misuse services have benefited from the national strategy set out in *Tackling Drugs to Build a Better Britain: The Government's 10-Year Strategy for Tackling Drug Misuse* (Cabinet Office 1998). However, to date the majority of available resources have been allocated to schemes working in tandem with the criminal justice system. With the current agenda to expand the capacity of substance misuse services (by 66% by 2005 and by 100% by 2008, UKADCU 2000), there is currently limited scope to develop whole new integrated treatment teams. Such dual diagnosis teams, as advocated by many of the experts from the United States, would not replicate existing secondary services and would create a considerable resource burden. This chapter aims to describe ways of responding to dual diagnosis effectively, utilising both existing health and social services resources in the UK. For a definition of terms used in the chapter see Table 7.1.

Table 7.1 Operational definitions

Term	Definition
Dual diagnosis	Describes the coexistence of mental illness and substance misuse
Consecutive treatment	Treatment programmes are delivered by the substance misuse team or mental health team depending on the presenting problem
Parallel treatment	Treatment is delivered by both the substance misuse team and the mental health team concurrently
Integrated treatment	A single treatment system (or dual diagnosis team) whereby the person's substance misuse and mental illness are treated simultaneously by the same clinician
Shared care	The delivery of parallel treatment with close collaboration and communication between teams and careful timing of interventions

Need for inter-agency collaboration

People with a lifetime history of schizophrenia in the United States are 4.6 times more likely to have a substance use disorder than the general population (Regier *et al.* 1990). A survey of comorbid substance misuse among people with psychotic illness in a British suburban setting reported a prevalence of 33% (Wright *et al.* 2000). These figures suggest that community mental health teams (CMHTs) have an important role to play in the holistic care of their client group. Appropriate interventions include harm reduction, early and brief interventions and systematic treatment for those with substance dependence and mental health problems (Pols *et al.* 1996). Unfortunately though, in many cases, there is reluctance on the part of CMHTs to become involved in the management of substance misuse by their patients. Unnithan *et al.* (1994) identified three areas of concern among general psychiatrists leading to a reluctance to address substance misuse in their patients:

(1) *Role adequacy*: having the necessary information and skills in order to screen and provide appropriate treatment.

(2) *Role legitimacy*: whether the management of substance misuse falls within their area of responsibility.

(3) *Role support*: the confidence that there is adequate advice and back-up of specialist services.

A recent survey of 143 psychiatrists in the UK reported that the majority had identified at least one new case of alcohol (61%) and drug misuse (55%) in the previous month. Less than half of the respondents had received formal training in the management of substance misuse in the previous five years. Despite this, there was general agreement about the potential management role for the doctor in the field (Day *et al.* 1999). This apparent willingness by psychiatrists to incorporate the management of substance misuse into existing roles does not detract from the need to address the educational deficit and to explore ways of facilitating a cooperative relationship between CMHTs and community drug and alcohol teams (CDATs).

The issue of dual diagnosis is very serious and causes profound problems for individuals, families and communities. It is now well understood that the misuse of drugs and/or alcohol by severely mentally ill people results in a poorer prognosis and may significantly increase the risk they pose to themselves or others. In this context, *Building Bridges: a guide to arrangements for inter-agency working for the care and protection of severely mentally ill people* (Department of Health 1996) was published. This document makes explicit the need for close links between CMHTs and CDATs to be maintained at provider level to ensure that care is properly coordinated. The framework for such a collaborative approach is set out through the application of the Care Programme Approach (CPA) (Department of Health 1990). The Care Programme Approach applies to all mentally ill patients who are accepted by mental health services. The essential elements of the CPA are:

- systematic assessment of health and social care needs;
- an agreed care plan allocation of a key worker/care co-ordinator; and
- regular review of the patient's progress.

Utilising such an approach makes clear the individual professional's responsibilities in the overall care plan. Multidisciplinary and multi-agency communication through participation at care planning and review meetings and circulation of the CPA documentation ensures coordination of care. While these arrangements can enhance shared care in theory, in practice philosophical differences and conflict between clinicians and teams will undermine them. The nature of these problems and strategies to assist in overcoming them will be set out. In the case of patients with severe mental illness, the key worker will normally be from the CMHT. The nature and timing of input from the CDAT can be discussed and agreed within the care planning meeting. Such an approach needs to be designed in a flexible, patient centred rather than programme centred way. The interventions need to be tailored to the individual patient's needs. Drake *et al.* (1993) described nine principles in the treatment of drug misuse in the severely mentally ill. They are:

(1) Assertive outreach
(2) Close monitoring
(3) Integration (or collaborative shared care)
(4) Comprehensiveness
(5) Stable living situation
(6) Flexibility
(7) Stage-wise treatment
(8) Longitudinal perspective
(9) Optimism.

These principles are sensitive to the fact that the severely mentally ill do not identify substance misuse problems and seek help in the way expected of others. They do not respond well to traditional addictions services which put the emphasis on motivation to engage and remain in treatment. While Drake and colleagues developed these ideas as the principles that underpin integrated treatment teams, they are equally applicable as principles to guide practice delivered through simultaneous, coordinated delivery of interventions by more than one team. All of the principles are within the scope of combined efforts but the key to success lies in effective joint working, communication and a shared vision.

Problems with inter-agency collaboration

Many will be familiar with the scenario whereby an individual presents to one service with psychotic and substance misuse problems. He or she is then redirected towards another team after the problem has been relabelled, and 'primary' status is given to the element of the problem that is not perceived to fall within the team's remit (Cantwell & Harrison 1996). Cyclical debates between clinicians from CDATs and CMHTs over what problem is primary and which team has medical responsibility for the patient is divisive. It tends to lead to disharmony at best and a complete break down in coworking at worst. The effect on patient care can be disastrous as it leads to sequential treatment delivery and poor interteam communication. A retrospective review of care collaboration and continuity was carried out on the records of 34 young people who had committed suicide (Wasserman 1998). It was found that poor continuity of care was a common feature. The case notes revealed that drug and alcohol misuse may have been noted, but the person's social problems tended to be identified as the only problem. Psychiatric problems were not detected and staff therefore found it difficult to offer appropriate treatment options. Poorly coordinated moves between treatment teams resulted in the main interruptions to continuity.

There are many reasons why historically CMHTs and CDATs have not formed effective partnerships. Wallen and Weiner (1989) identified a number of impediments to a collaborative approach by CMHTs. These include the premature diagnosis of a psychiatric disorder based on the behavioural symptoms of substance misuse, ignorance, fear and a lack of knowledge of chemical dependency and simplistic approaches (e.g. 'just say no'). However, Gafoor and Rassool (1998) point out that mental health nurses do possess the core therapeutic skills to work with substance misusers. But they may be reluctant to intervene due to low confidence in their ability to facilitate change in their client's substance use or they may hold negative views towards the outcome of their interventions.

Further reasons why closer cooperation between mental health and substance misuse teams is difficult because they are often functionally, administratively and geographically separated (Kavanagh *et al.* 2000). The two systems operate with different treatment philosophies. Though many professionals within the substance misuse treatment setting have a background in psychiatry, their professional lives often diverge from their counterparts in adult general psychiatry (Allen & Gerace 1996). The emotive response to substance misuse occasionally encountered by some in adult psychiatry becomes a further impediment. Despite both disorders being viewed as aetiologically multifactorial, it is rare for a person with a mental health problem to be viewed as having 'brought it on themself', but this has been the response to inaction on the part of clinicians when substance misuse is encountered.

Within the mental health field there continue to be difficulties in enabling professional groups to work effectively together within teams, so it is hardly surprising that collaborative work between teams poses further problems. The reasons for poor interprofessional teamwork highlighted by Roberts and Priest (1997) are consistent with the difficulties encountered in the care of those with dual diagnosis. They include:

- rigid role demarcation;
- professional elitism;
- vested professional interest;
- poor communications; and
- misunderstandings about responsibilities.

Even in cases where both teams become concurrently involved in the care of an individual patient, each clinician's treatment outcome expectation can be a barrier to effective treatment. Abstinence may be perceived as the only desirable outcome by the CMHT, and the CDAT may take the view they can only intervene if the psychiatric symptomatology is absent. Clearly, for concurrent treatment to take place there needs to be dialogue and agreement that a reduction/change in use of substances is the appropriate way forward, and abstinence, however, desirable, may not be realistic. A reduction in the use of substances may improve psychiatric symptomatology directly or increase treatment compliance. Even so, psychosocial interventions for patients in the precontemplative phase of the cycle of change, including cognitive therapy (e.g. motivational interviewing) can be incorporated into the treatment of patients suffering from psychotic illness and substance misuse (Swanson *et al.* 1999). In this way, a more realistic appraisal of treatment outcome expectation can enable a symbiotic approach from each service.

Gilvary (1998) points out that the coordination of services and treatment philosophies and the timing of interventions are more important than the integration of staff. This is the very heart of the matter. While integrated treatment systems or dual diagnosis teams may be a helpful, if unproven model, providing a coordinated response in areas where there is a high prevalence of comorbidity (some inner city areas with significant social deprivation). They are not a realistic response in most localities. Therefore the challenges are first to explore how services can respond collaboratively to effectively meet the need of those with dual diagnosis and second how can diverse treatment philosophies become harmonious and patient centred as regards dual diagnosis.

Overcoming the barriers

Those working in the field will probably be only too familiar with the tendency to lack of cooperation and partnership working between substance misuse services and mental health teams. There is a pressing need for a greater recognition of psychiatric problems and comorbidity by all professionals, both specialist and generic (Gilvary 1998).

In the long term, to undermine this polarised response to issues of comorbidity, the whole issue of the misuse of substances needs to be integrated far more extensively into the undergraduate and postgraduate training programmes of mental health professionals (Crome 1999; Royal College of Psychiatrists 2000). There also needs to be a concerted research programme to determine the most effective model of service delivery before considerable investment is made in a model driven by expediency rather than by an evidence base (Weaver *et al.* 1999). In the short and medium term, due to the problems described, existing services must be enabled to meet the demands and find ways to work together. Ideally, mental health teams would manage the misuse of substances by their patients and substance misuse teams would address the mental health problems manifested by their patients. However in the real world, the dynamic nature of these interrelated problems, on a continuum of severity, means that at times, a particularly specialist collaborative response is called for. In the UK we have well established sector CMHTs. Johnson (1997) argues for substance misuse treatment to be integrated into these teams through developing existing services rather than establishing new ones. Three potential service developments are suggested:

(1) The attachment of an addictions professional to each sector team facilitating referrals and joint discussion;

(2) A specialist dual diagnosis worker to be attached to each community team; and

(3) Provision of additional training and supervision in addiction techniques for all CMHT staff.

The appointment of an addictions professional for each sector CMHT would be likely to fail due to financial and recruitment problems. The provision of the dual diagnosis worker may have the effect of psychologically absolving the CDAT and other CMHT staff of responsibility for this group. The dual diagnosis worker will clearly be unable to take on the target group which is known to constitute 33–47% of those with severe mental illness (Regier *et al.* 1990; Menezes *et al.* 1996; Wright *et al.* 2000). The provision of training and supervision to CMHT staff is very important. However it does not fully utilise the skills of specialist addiction clinicians and is therefore only one element of a collaborative interagency programme.

Much has been written about ineffective collaborative interventions for dual diagnosis. One example of effective inter-agency collaborative working is reported by Ridgley *et al.* (1998). She describes an innovative programme to empower existing services rather than establish new, expensive dual diagnosis teams. To improve the diagnosis and treatment of people with dual diagnosis four regional collaboratives were established in the state of Maine in the US. These comprised representatives from mental health, public health and substance abuse treatment providers, service users, families and other organisations. The major focus was to build provider relationships across service sector boundaries, establish a common language to communicate about diagnosis and treatment and to provide inter-agency training. A survey of one of the collaboratives, at one and two years, revealed an increase in inter-agency referrals, joint assessments of clients, inter-agency training and joint sponsorship of specific client treatment programmes. These findings support the view that where a collaborative approach has been organised in response to dual diagnosis, the professional relationships that develop between services form the basis for sustained inter-agency working. Rodgers (1994) states, 'to pursue and achieve interprofessional collaboration, professionals need to value their sense of worth and relinquish defensiveness'. In order to realise this statement, CMHT staff and CDAT staff need first to be clear about their role and second to be clear about the role of others. Resistance to interteam collaboration by individuals will need to be explored within the context of clinical supervision and worked through in a supported manner. There may be issues of transference that relate to past experience or conflicts. Such issues need to be addressed and not avoided. Resistant individuals can have an undermining effect on team morale and can be unconsciously divisive.

Local strategies to develop new systems

Organising existing service structures to respond to the needs of those with comorbid problems in a timely manner can be achieved in several ways. First there can be an encouragement of arrangements for members of both the substances misuse team and mental health team to develop a particular interest in the issue of comorbidity and act as a liaison between teams. The training of these individuals can be focused in such a way so they become a source of information and supervision for their colleagues. Furthermore they can link with their counterpart in the opposite team and collaborate when people with comorbid problems are referred to their teams. In this way, professionals can work beyond agency boundaries and form 'logical teams' defined by the professionals and workers on the patient's care plan or CPA documentation and not solely by the agency structure. The adoption of more flexible, whole systems way of working, operating across organisational boundaries, is alien to traditional bureaucratic practice endemic in so many statutory services. It is however, in keeping with the spirit of *Tackling Drugs to Build a Better Britain* (Cabinet Office 1998), and *Building Bridges* (Department of Health 1996), which have inter-agency collaboration and cooperation at their core. It also places the patient's needs rather than the service's custom and practice as the driver for care planning. The therapeutic response is designed to fit the patient rather than attempting to fit the patient to the service. The team's custom and practice will then adapt to align with good practice.

This is all very well, but it does not address the problem where there are difficulties in working relationships between two teams. These problems often occur in the context of a history of conflict, and a culture of silence or antagonism can result. The response to this situation may be from a managerial or 'shop floor' level but the latter may be more effective. A will to alter the situation at some level is the only prerequisite for change. This may have to come from a managerial or senior level within one of the disciplines. Strategies to address such difficulties have been described in texts on working with diversity within whole systems approaches (Pratt *et al.* 1999). The driver for change needs to come from the manipulation of key individuals within the whole system (e.g. the NHS Trust). Barriers to collaboration are as much about an organisational as practitioner culture (Trevillion 1995). Change results from supporting new connections between people to challenge and influence a maladaptive situation through the development of a counterculture. The mix of people within such a group should include carefully identified change agents (Pratt *et al.* 1999):

• different levels of clinicians from both teams and from within the organisation

• people who know how 'to connect' and are interested in doing things differently (some of whom may be 'troublesome')

• the sort of people whose support makes it likely that others will follow.

Bringing together groups of such people within an organisation, with the aim of analysing the problems with interteam collaboration and exploring how shared care for dual diagnosis can be approached is the first step in the management of change. Closer intersectoral communication can be further facilitated through reviewing confidentiality policies. The necessary climate for shared care is enabled by sharing patient information appropriately, taking into account the advice of the professional bodies and the Data Protection Act. Exchanging client information and holding joint case conferences facilitates the development of shared treatment plans in the spirit of the CPA. Kavanagh *et al.* (2000) recommend further collaborative advances such as offering consultation facilities within team bases and conducting joint assessments. Working in this way engenders a culture of working together towards a common goal rather than adopting a territorial position leading to compartmentalised care.

Conducting joint assessments enables each clinician to observe each other assessment process. This presents an advantage at several levels. First, it exposes each clinician to a clinical situation with a true shared agenda that may assist in changing opposing team philosophies. Second, it presents an important learning opportunity enabling the sharing of skills and assessment styles. Finally, it forms the basis of clear communication between clinicians so there is mutual understanding about clinical responsibility and roles in the care of the patient. Through the practical experience of joint assessments and shared care, clinicians from each team are more likely to be able to develop a sense of understanding that is difficult in the absence of first hand experience of working with this client group. It is therefore likely that individuals within teams become apparent who are able to develop an interest in taking a more leading role in the care of patients with dual diagnosis. Such people are those who can develop liaison roles as already described, and may also coordinate a programme of reciprocal teaching and learning in theory and practice. Such educational initiatives can bring about a greater understanding of the technical aspects of each professional's speciality and work towards engendering a sense of team empathic understanding of the key issues and challenges. Collaborative assessment and education will both enhance quality of care and be protective against future interteam disputes.

Treatment adherence is one of the major challenges facing those working with patients with severe mental illness and more particularly with patients with dual diagnosis. There is evidence that motivational interviewing (Miller & Rollnick 1991) which is a cognitive behavioural intervention almost universally applied within the addictions field, can significantly improve outpatient treatment adherence among psychiatric and dually diagnosed patients (Swanson *et al.* 1999). Those working in the addiction field with skills in the delivery of motivational interviewing represent an important information and training resource for those working in general adult psychiatry. Sharing of such advances in theory and practice and by exploring ways in which teams can work together towards a common goal are important steps towards more effectively meeting the needs of those with dual diagnosis.

Conclusion

The issue of dual diagnosis is one of the most pressing issues presently facing the fields of substance misuse and mental health. It is being poorly addressed in most localities, and there are examples of reluctance on the part of some clinicians to become more involved. With the current (June 2001) government's drugs agenda to address links between drug misuse and crime and the drive to capacity build, the scope to initiate new service structures is limited. The challenge is therefore how to enable existing services to address dual diagnosis more effectively through a sharing of knowledge, skills and patient care. Training is central to the long-term strategy to overcome the problems in service delivery for this group. Curriculum planners need to incorporate content on dual diagnosis into undergraduate and postgraduate training programmes in the caring professions. At a local level there need to be programmes of reciprocal training between teams coordinated by clinicians with an interest and training in the issue of dual diagnosis. Where there is resistance to collaboration between teams, organisations have a responsibility to address this comprehensively. Team resistance needs to be addressed through change management strategies, identifying the change agents and altering the mix of individuals within teams. However, the organisational culture may be at the root of the problem. Resistance by individuals needs to be addressed through training and clinical supervision. The development of informal link/liaison roles between CMHTs and CDATs can assist in enabling interteam communication by providing a point of contact for clinicians from each team. These individuals can act as a source of information and supervision for colleagues, ensuring they are not seen as the 'dual diagnosis worker' for the team.

The CPA provides the framework for effective collaboration between teams. It formalises shared care arrangements and helps to ensure patients with dual diagnosis do not fall between two teams. There is a statutory requirement to apply CPA to patients taken on by psychiatric teams, and this has a particular relevance in dual diagnosis cases where poor treatment compliance and risk to self and colleagues are more likely than in the broader general adult psychiatric population. The nine principles of treatment for dual diagnosis described by Drake *et al.* (1993) can be applied in shared care working for the group. They underpin good practice and the inclusion of joint assessments and care planning means the integration described by Drake is incorporated in the absence of a single treatment modality. The inclusion of motivational interviewing into the treatment repertoire for this group by CMHTs will bring evidenced based practice into clinical practice. While this chapter has described ways of enabling existing CDATs and CMHTs to become more effective in their response to dual diagnosis there is still a resource issue. The training proposed and the development of liaison roles cannot occur unless commissioners and managers recognise that these initiatives require investment. If this is the case, there is cause for optimism.

References

Allen, K.M. & Gerace, L.M. (1996) Psychiatric nursing. In: K.M. Allen (ed.) *Nursing Care of the Addicted Client*. Lippincott-Raven, Philadelphia.

Cabinet Office (1998) *Tackling Drugs to Build a Better Britain: The Government's 10-Year Strategy for Tackling Drug Misuse*. Crown Copyright. ISBN 0101394527.

Cantwell, R. & Harrison, G. (1996) Substance misuse in the severely mentally ill. *Advances in Psychiatric Treatment* **2**, 117–124.

Crome, I.B. (1999) The trouble with training: substance misuse training in British medical schools revisited. What are the issues? *Drugs: Education, Prevention and Policy* **6**, 111–123.

Day, E., Arcelus, J. & Kahn, A. (1999) Perceived role of psychiatrists in the management of substance misuse: A questionnaire survey. *Psychiatric Bulletin* **23** (11), 667–670.

Department of Health (1990) *Caring for People. Care Programme Approach for People with a Mental Illness Referred to the Special Psychiatric Services*. HMSO, London.

Department of Health (1996) *Building Bridges: a guide to arrangements for inter-agency working for the care and protection of severely mentally ill people*. Department of Health, Wetherby.

Department of Health (1999) *Safer Services: National Confidential Inquiry into Suicide and Homicide by People with Mental Illness*. Department of Health, London.

Drake, R.E., Bartels, S.J., Teagues, G.B., Noordsy, D.L. & Clark, R.E. (1993) Treatment of substance abuse in severely mentally ill patients. *Journal of Nervous and Mental Disease*. **181**, 606–611.

Drake, R.E., Mercer-McFadden, C., Mueser, K.T., McHugo, G.J. & Bond, G.R. (1998) Review of integrated mental health and substance abuse treatment for patients with dual disorders. *Schizophrenia Bulletin* **24** (4), 589–608.

Gafoor, M. & Rassool, G. Hussein (1998) The co-existence of psychiatric disorders and substance misuse: working with dual diagnosis patients. *Journal of Advanced Nursing* **27**, 497–502.

George, T.P. & Krystal, J.H. (2000) Comorbidity of psychiatric and substance misuse disorders. *Current Opinion in Psychiatry* **13**, 327–331.

Gilvary, E. (1998) Psychiatric perspective: relationship between psychiatric and psychological disorders and symptomatology. In: R. Robertson (ed.) *Management of Drug Users in the Community.* Arnold, London.

Johnson, S. (1997) Dual diagnosis of severe mental illness and substance misuse: a case for specialist services? *British Journal of Psychiatry* **171**, 205–208.

Kavanagh, D.J., Greenaway, L., Jenner, L., Saunders, J.B., White, A., Sorban, J. & Hamilton, G. (2000) Contrasting views and experiences of health professionals on the management of comorbid substance misuse and mental disorders. *Australian and New Zealand Journal of Psychiatry* **34**, 279–289.

Ley, A., Jeffrey, D.P., McLaren, S. & Siegfried, N. (2000) Treatment programmes for people with both severe mental illness and substance misuse. Cochrane Database of Systematic Reviews [computer file]. (2): CD001088.

Menezes, P.R., Johnson, S., Thornicroft, G., Marshall, J., Prossor, D., Bebbington, P. & Kuipers, E. (1996) Drug and alcohol problems among individuals with severe mental illness in South London. *British Journal of Psychiatry* **168**, 612–619.

Miller, W.R. & Rollnick, S. (1991) *Motivational Interviewing: Preparing People to Change Addictive Behaviour.* Guilford Press, New York.

Mueser, K.T., Drake, R.E. & Noordsy, D.L. (1998) Integrated mental health and substance abuse treatment for severe psychiatric disorders. *Journal of Practice Psychiatry and Behavioural Health* **May**, 129–139.

Pols, R.G., Sellman, D., Jurd, S., Baigent, M., Waddy, N., Sacks, T., Tucker, P., Fowler, J. & White, A. (1996) What is the psychiatrist's role in drugs and alcohol? *Australian and New Zealand Journal of Psychiatry* **30** (4), 540–548.

Pratt, J., Gordon, P. & Plamping, D. (1999) *Working Whole Systems. Putting Theory into Practice in Organisations.* Kings Fund, London.

Regier, D.A., Farmer, M.E., Rae, D.S., Locke, B.Z., Keith, S.J., Judd, L.L. & Goodwin, F.K. (1990) Comorbidity of mental disorders with alcohol and other drug abuse. Results from the Epidemiological Catchment Area (ECA) study. *JAMA* **264**, 2511–2518.

Ridgley, M.S., Lambert, D., Goodman, A., Chichester, C.S. & Ralph, R. (1998) Interagency collaboration in services for people with co-occurring mental illness and substance use disorder. *Psychiatric Services* **49**, 236–238.

Roberts, P. & Priest, H. (1997) Achieving interprofessional working in mental health. *Nursing Standard* **12** (2), 39–41.

Rodgers, J. (1994) Collaboration among health professionals. *Nursing Standard* **9** (6), 25–26.

Royal College of Psychiatrists (2000) *Drugs: Dilemmas and Choices.* Gaskell, London.

Swanson, A.J., Pantalon, M.V. & Cohen, K.R. (1999) Motivational interviewing and treatment adherence among psychiatric and dually diagnosed patients. *Journal of Nervous and Mental Disease* **87** (10), 630–635.

Trevillion, S. (1995) Competence to collaborate. *CAIPE Bulletin* **10**, 6.

United Kingdom Anti-Drug Co-ordinator's Unit (UKADCU) (2000) *Second National Plan 2000/2001.* Cabinet Office, London.

Unnithan, S., Ritson, B. & Strang, J. (1994) Organising treatment services for drug and alcohol misusers. In: J. Chick & R. Cantwell (eds) *Seminars in Alcohol and Drug Misusers.* Gaskell, London, pp. 223–238.

Wallen, M. & Weiner, H. (1989) The dually diagnosed patient in an in patient chemical dependency treatment program. *Alcoholism Treatment Quarterly* **5** (1/2), 197–218.

Wasserman, H.A. (1998) Lack of continuity—a problem in the care of young suicides. *Acta Psychiatrica Scandinavica* **97**, 326–333.

Weaver, T., Renton, A., Stimson, G. & Tyrer, P. (1999) Severe mental illness and substance misuse. *British Medical Journal* **318**, 137–138.

Wright, S., Gournay, K., Glorney, E. & Thornicroft, G. (2000) Dual diagnosis in the suburbs: prevalence, need and in-patient service use. *Social Psychiatry and Psychiatric Epidemiology* **35** (7), 297–304.

8: A Synthesis of Addiction & Mental Health Nursing: An Approach to Community Interventions

Kim Moore and G. Hussein Rassool

Introduction

Dual diagnosis is not a new phenomenon, a growing interest in the comorbidity of individuals with a mental health problem and substance misuse problem began to focus in the early 1980s. Since the mid 1990s, in the United Kingdom (UK), there has been considerable interest by addiction nurses and mental health professionals in the care and management of mentally ill patients who misuse psychoactive substances. The White paper *Tackling Drugs to Build a Better Britain* (Cabinet Office 1998) identified links between substance misuse and mental health problems for the first time. Assertive outreach became an identified focus for treatment strategies, and following the release of *Tackling Drugs to Build a Better Britain*, funding for dual diagnosis services was made available through specific grant projects (Sainsbury's Centre for Mental Health 1998). The National Service Framework for Mental Health (NSF 2000) and Drug Action Team guidance (2000) clearly identify dual diagnosis patients as a population with higher rates of illness and a greater risk of stigmatisation and exclusion from existing service provision. The development of community based practices targeting vulnerable groups such as dual diagnosis have been outlined in Standard One of the NSF, such practices are beginning to evolve in selected locations in the UK.

The term dual diagnosis has been coined to describe patients with coexistent mental illness and substance misuse problems (Carey *et al.* 1991). Some mentally ill patients may self medicate their symptoms with illicit drugs and alcohol and others, receiving neuroleptic medication, may use stimulant type drugs to counteract distressing extra-pyramidal side-effects (Schneider & Siris 1987; Dixon *et al.* 1990). In the UK, with the closures of long-stay psychiatric institutions and an increasing emphasis on care and treatment in the community, mentally ill patients are perhaps more exposed to a range of licit and illicit drugs than previously. Furthermore, mentally ill people who have become socially isolated, may be drawn into a drug using subculture that appears more attractive and less stigmatised for social interactions (Gafoor &

Rassool 1998). The failure to recognise mental health problems among sub-stance misusers and vice versa can lead to ineffective management and treat-ment outcomes. Even when a diagnosis problem is identified, many patients tend to fall between the substance misuse services and mental health agen-cies with both respectively operating separately and under different philoso-phies and treatment regimes (Gafoor & Rassool 1998).

Because of the close involvement of addiction nurses and mental health nurses with patients in both residential and community settings, they are in a unique position to develop effective interventions and management strategies for dual diagnosis patients. However, a survey by McKeown and Liebling (1995) showed that awareness of the problems of dual diagnosis among mental health nurses was low. Nurses may be reluctant to intervene with substance misuse problems either due to lack of knowledge and exper-tise regarding substance misuse or having negative attitudes towards the substance misuser. Mental health nurses consider those with substance use problems difficult to treat and addiction nurses feel that they are not pre-pared to work with psychiatric patients (Allen & Gerace 1996). In effect, most addiction nurses are trained in mental health nursing in the UK. However, overtly self-abusive behaviour particularly when it involves illicit drugs, can be dealt with in a suppressive and moralist way by many health care workers not least of all nurses, probably out of a sense of frustration or inadequacy about an ability to effect any change (Gafoor 1985). Rassool (2000) asserted that among health care professionals dealing with substance misuse and mental health problems there may be dissonance between their personal belief—therapeutic pessimism, that is there is nothing that can be done or should be done—and their professional roles (de-skilled, lacking in confidence etc.).

It would be compelling to raise both the awareness of nurses and others and to provide adequate preparation in areas of substance misuse and men-tal health problems. However, it is argued that at present, much professional education and training of health care professionals reinforces the view that dealing with substance misuse is a specialist's job (Rassool 1993).

The aims of this chapter are to outline the development of community oriented services for dual diagnosis patients and examine some of the para-meters of addiction nursing. It will also address the role of nurses and spe-cialist workers and the implications of dual diagnosis education and training for nurses.

Development of community oriented services

Community nursing in dual diagnosis originates within the United States of America (US), with established community programmes ranging from out-patient services to specialist outreach services. The US leads the way with dedicated research, developing separate funding streams for specific treat-ment of dual diagnosis patients from hospital to community settings. One key feature of the programmes developed for community interventions is the research into the needs of the local population, evaluating the efficacy of the programmes offered, joint working, training and research (Zweeben 1993; Siegfried *et al.* 1999). However, there is no conclusive evidence that gives a blueprint to service provision, or supports any best approach of meeting the needs of complex care, dual diagnosis or coexisting substance misuse problems. Evidence from the US suggests small caseloads, relapse prevention techniques, assertive outreach, financial management schemes and social interventions can influence the number of admissions to acute or crisis facilities (Osher & Kofoed 1989). Thus, reducing the potential for dual diagnosis patients to fall between the service provisions.

In the UK, health and social care policies implemented by the government coupled with the changing health care needs of the population have provided added impetus in the care and management of a significant proportion of the population with substance misuse and mental health problems. Community oriented services for substance misusers and mental health problems emerged from this sociocultural and political shift. The number of statutory and non-statutory addictions agencies, which previously excluded mental health, are now working with dual diagnosis patients. Services being developed in the UK show their origins in programmes developed in New Hampshire, US (Osher & Kofoed 1989). This broadly includes the development of specialist dual diagnosis teams working within both substance misuse and mental health, individual liaison staff within Community Mental Health Teams (CMHTs) and community drug and alcohol agencies or staff who provide training for mental health teams about substance misuse.

Regardless of the model chosen by a service, criticisms can be levelled to the duplication of work, lack of clarity around the responsibility of care provision. In addition, the separation of the user group from established support systems can create greater prejudices about the nature of dual diagnosis and willingness for working in partnership (Thacker & Tremaine 1989). Specialist dual diagnosis services are being developed within the UK, varying widely in their approaches. Multidisciplinary teams that are client orientated, with allocated client caseloads can be found, alongside the utilisation of the liaison, consultation and training models. Other organisations have appointed a single individual, who may act as a facilitator or educator to both addictions and mental health services. The care programme approach formalised levels of responsibility for the Community Psychiatric Nurses. This is not so for addictions, where the patient is seen to be responsible and accountable for their actions. Dual diagnosis nursing combines the core principle of mental health by actively intervening to prevent active harm to self and others, whilst balancing this against the responsibilities of the patient for their actions. This is a fine boundary, and there is no definitive formula to assist with making a balanced decision. Such dichotomy of roles outlines one of the principle difficulties of working in dual diagnosis — how to bridge this gap and achieve a balance between the two divergent philosophies.

Addiction nursing as a speciality

Historically, occupational labels such as alcohol nurse, drug dependency nurse, chemical substance nurse, specialist nurse in addiction and community psychiatric nurse (addiction) have been ascribed to those working with substance misusers (Rassool 1997). It was not until the mid 1980s that addiction nursing as a clinical speciality, within the broader framework of mental health nursing, began to put its clinical and academic roots. Addiction nursing may be defined as a specialist branch of mental health nursing concerned with the care and treatment interventions aimed at those individuals whose health problems are directly related to the use and misuse of psychoactive substances and to other addictive behaviours such as eating disorders and gambling (Rassool 1997). It is argued that, although the concept of addiction nursing may be criticised on the grounds that it is too medically orientated and substance focused, other ascribed labels are too generic and lack the distinctive professional representation of addiction nursing (Rassool 1997). Thus, the scope of professional practice in addiction nursing and mental health nursing incorporates the activities of clinical practice nursing, a range of psychosocial intervention strategies including complementary therapies), education, policy-making, research and all other pursuits through which nurse practitioners contribute to the care and in the interests of the clients.

Addiction nurses practise in both residential and community settings and have an excellent track record in developing innovative health care initiatives and community-oriented programmes for substance misusers and many of the key developments in recent years have been nurse-led. These include smoking cessation clinics, mobile methadone clinics, outreach work with drug using prostitutes, and satellite clinics for homeless drinkers and development of multi-professional postgraduate educational programmes in addictive behaviour (Rassool & Gafoor 1997; Rassool 2000). The massive expansion of community services for substance misusers such as the development of community drug/alcohol teams, drug alcohol liaison teams, day care programmes, street agencies, outreach work and needle exchange schemes has heralded the potential development of addiction nursing as a community speciality (Rassool 1999).

Commonalities and differences in nursing roles

There are more commonalities than differences in the nursing roles of the addiction nurses and mental health nurses. The primary role of addiction nurses or mental health nurses exemplifies the contribution that they can make to comprehensive patient care by performing clinical interventions from triage to counselling, psychotherapy to case management (Greenman 1994). Due to the nature of the work and the composition of many community mental health teams and community drug and alcohol teams, the blurring of roles among the disciplines is highly apparent. Much of the everyday work with substance misusers involves certain care skills for example, assessment, counselling and relapse prevention, and decisions regarding whether a client is seen by a nurse, medical practitioner or psychologist have, in the past, often depended upon which discipline was in charge of the allocation process and which staff member had a vacant slot (Gafoor 1997). This phenomenon is no different in community mental health teams.

A comparison of the primary roles within mental health and substance misuse is shown in Table 8.1 which highlights many of the similarities for each discipline. There are considerable number of transferable roles and skills that are shared between mental health and addiction nursing that can be combined to enable effective nursing within dual diagnosis populations. Dual diagnosis nursing can thus be seen as a synthesis of principles of care and management from both addiction and mental health fields.

Nurses provide comprehensive and ongoing assessments in all aspects of their work, in dual diagnosis, the clinical work is dependent on broad nurs-

Table 8.1 Comparison of nursing roles

	Psychiatric nursing	Addiction nursing	Dual diagnosis nursing
Assessment	Concerned primarily with mental health presentation • Presenting factors history of presenting factors • Treatment compliance • Section of mental health act including specialist assessments such as forensic and eating disorders • Risk to self and others • Level of insight into mental health • Current mood • Current behaviour • Use of psychotropic medications • Use of drugs and alcohol • Brief intervention • Motivational interviewing	Concerned primarily with illicit drug use • Drug/s of choice • Amount and frequency • Risks around substance misuse • Risk related to behaviours to support substance misuse • Level of insight into substance use and effects of use • Motivations to change • Relapse prevention	Concerned with substance misuse in the presenting mental health • Drug/s of choice currently used, including psychotropic medications • Amount and frequency of substance misuse • History of substance misuse in relation to occurrence of psychiatric symptoms • Risks related to the use of drugs and alcohol, including the implication for harm to self or others and risk behaviours related to obtaining drugs or alcohol • Level of insight to both mental health and substance misuse • Current mood • Current behaviour • Motivation for change
Medication	Concerned with psychotropic medications • Effects • Side-effects • Overdose • Actions and interactions • Supervised consumption • Administration of depot medications • Medication compliance	Concerned with illicit and licit substances, including prescription medications • Effects of drugs and alcohol • Side-effects of drugs and alcohol • Withdrawal effects of drugs and alcohol • Overdose and accidental overdose	Concerned with psychotropic and prescribed medications • Effects of illicit substances and prescribed medications • Actions and interactions of prescribed and non-prescribed medications • Side-effects of both substances of abuse and prescribed medications • Overdose and accidental overdose

Table 8.1 (*Continued*)

	Psychiatric nursing	Addiction nursing	Dual diagnosis nursing
		• Supervised consumption of methadone • Administration of detoxification medications • Additional substance misuse during substitute prescribing	• Administration of medication for detoxification • Supervised consumption of methadone • Medication compliance, including additional substance use during substitute prescribing
Health checks	• Weight • Height • Urine testing for basic analysis • Sleep patterns • Dietary intake • Hygiene patterns	• Substance misuse either by urine testing or via breathalyser • Injecting sites for damage • Hepatitis and HIV testing can be offered • Requests for full blood counts/liver function tests and confirmation of substance misuse	• Weight • Height • Urine testing for basic analysis and substance misuse • Breath testing for alcohol use • Hygiene at initial presentation • Injection sites for damage • Dietary intake • Requests for full blood counts/ liver function tests and confirmation of substance misuse
Nursing care offered	• Risk assessments for harm to self and others • Ongoing mental health assessments • Active role in the Community Programme Approach • Key worker responsibility for out-patients • Administration of medications including depot medications • Individual counselling/ individual support/group work • Work on insight into mental health and development of strategies related to activities of daily living • Support of relatives/ partners and other family members • Development of structured programmes and care plans enhancing mental health • Simple wound dressings	• Supervision of methadone consumption and where applicable on site injecting clinics • Harm minimisation of substance use • Counselling specific to the use and reduction of drugs and alcohol • Supervision of home detoxification programmes • Administration of methadone prescriptions • Community care funding assessments for inpatient treatment • Simple wound dressings • Individual/group counselling	• Risk assessments for harm to self and others • Supervision of medications including methadone and psychotropic prescriptions • individuals supported counselling • Outreach work to enhance engagement within local services • Harm minimisation for substance misuse and harm to self or others • Counselling specific to mental health and substance misuse • Supervision of outpatient detoxification for substance misuse • Administration of methadone prescriptions • Adjunctive role in Community Programme Approach/ Community Care funding assessments • Development of care plans to optimise patient care • Simple wound dressings

These are comparisons of roles and not exhaustive lists.

ing skills. The art of completing a dual diagnosis assessment relies on incorporating two essential elements:

(1) level and nature of risks in evidence by the presenting patient/client; and

(2) history and current nature of the type and frequency of psychoactive substances used.

A central aspect of working in dual diagnosis is the ability to provide a comprehensive assessment of mental health history and current symptoms, current and historical substance use and misuse and current physical health and how these three major aspects impact on the current presentation or baseline behaviour. The assessment phase should also include observation for psychiatric symptoms relating to intoxication and withdrawal from various psychoactive substances (see Table 8.2). One feature of a dual diagnosis assessment is the use of 'time lines', by recording the sequence of events for both substance misuse and mental health problems over a given time period. Time lines can provide invaluable information, particularly in relation to which event occurs first, substance misuse or mental health, additionally they can be used to help indicate priority for treatment actions.

Evidence based practice requires that all formulations for nursing care are based on fact. In dual diagnosis, a combination of current behaviours, mood and physiological changes for both mental health and substance misuse enables comprehensive treatment programmes to be established. An additional requirement for nurses is the development of a working plan of action, as providers of care, skills such as basic drug and alcohol education, and the knowledge of how substance misuse interacts with, and affects mental health states is essential. Such individual care programme meets the criteria for CPA, and requires that nurses develop techniques that operate within different settings, and for many different levels of patient sophistication.

Other activities that can be considered include:

• Designing patient literature on basic psychiatry and addictions information.

• Support and advice for partners and parents.

• Development of literature on basic psychiatry/addictions for professional groups.

Table 8.2 A summary of assessment criteria for dual diagnosis

---

• Violence, homelessness, poor treatment compliance and repeated admissions are more common among mentally ill patient with a substance misuse disorder
• Physical examination, e.g. signs of injecting marks, enlarged liver
• Observation of mental health symptoms relating to intoxication and withdrawal of drugs and alcohol
• Collateral information from friends and relatives; and the use of toxicological screening
• Use of screening questionnaires
• Assessment of health care needs

- Involvement in patient support groups.
- Involvement in policy setting and review for mental health and addictions.

Nursing interventions within dual diagnosis populations are varied, falling broadly under three categories, medical/nursing practice, educational and psychotherapeutic interventions. Medically orientated practices such as urine testing, health checks, immunisations for hepatitis, detoxification from substances and supervision of prescribed medications such as methadone or psychotropic medications are all nursing roles.

Whilst some nursing interventions are predetermined by access to tools like breathalysers and rapid drug testing, the availability of information on local services, patient information and literature relating to drugs, alcohol and mental health is equally important. Inherent within nursing practice is the ability to educate. Dual diagnosis nursing embodies educational principles of harm minimisation by using a blend of addiction and mental health philosophies to determine individual practice. Such practice is exemplified in services that range from advice/information, counselling, health advice, group work to outreach and befriending strategies. Psychotherapeutic interventions by nursing staff can be found in the recognition of characteristics and consequences of substance misuse and mental health sequelae, with the implementation of nursing actions that addresses these consequences. Nurses have the ability to link this to the potential for the reduction of harm; as such these strategies are skilled interventions by nursing staff, and ones that are made on a daily basis.

Individual support programmes, psycho-dynamic and person-centred counselling, group work, motivational interviewing, brief interventions, to cognitive and behavioural programmes are some of the interventions offered by nurses. A central feature of dual diagnosis work in the community is the implementation of programmes within multidisciplinary teams, working with practitioners from primary health care teams, addiction teams or acute mental health teams to provide specialist care. This ensures there is support and expertise for working with this complex client group and demonstrates how nurses take important roles in the provision and coordination of care without working in isolation. Whilst there are no interventions specifically designed for working with dual diagnosis patients: there are also no barriers to utilising different interventions and innovations from other related fields.

Problems and issues

Patients with a coexisting mental health disorder and substance misuse problem present great challenges for nurses and other health care professionals. There are several problems and issues regarding the engagement and interventions of patients with dual diagnosis.

Many patients may have had difficulty engaging with psychiatric services due to substance use, or failed at the addictions treatment by defaulting on the prescribed programme. This group of patients are often thought of as 'difficult to treat', non-compliant or non-attenders. Patients often face the prejudice of having not just a mental health problem or substance misuse problem; they have both, and as such can be doubly rejected (National Service Framework for Mental Health 1999). There are additional prejudices that can add to this picture, ethnicity, culture, gender, education and social standing are factors that influence diagnosis and the perceived levels of risk made by professional groups. In working with the dual diagnosis population our own fears and prejudices about the complexity of the physical, emotional, moral and ethical problems must be examined.

In bridging the gap between mental health and substance misuse it is common to encounter the difficult area of 'responsibility' and 'confidentiality'. Dual diagnosis teams run the risk of being seen to be ultimately responsible for all dual diagnosis clients, whether they are appropriate for either addictions or mental health services or not. Abdication of responsibility for this client group can be due to concerns of risk, and an inability to deal with the duality of the presenting problems, or lack of expertise with this complex client group. Risk has been highlighted as a growing concern within community nursing management of dual diagnosis. Recent literature has suggested that dual diagnosis patients are regarded as high-risk patients for violence, and criminal behaviour, and even in homicides (Ward & Applin 1998; Scott *et al*. 1999). It is understandable that many practitioners have concerns in working with this client group. However, the obstacles must balance information on violence, fear and sometimes prejudice from systems that exclude them from engaging. While it can be argued that the nature of dual diagnosis may compound the level of risk, the full extent of violent behaviour and dual diagnosis continue to be assessed. Clinical practice of risk management at service level remains a thorny issue, a combination of mental health and substance misuse risk assessments would be important components of any comprehensive dual diagnosis work. Community nursing of this client group requires that in a similar vein to community mental health, safety is one of the most important components of day-to-day working, regardless which model the dual diagnosis service is based on.

Confidentiality as a core principal service provision continues to remain a difficult issue for health care professionals and substance misuse services, who have a long history of strict guidelines on both confidentiality and breach of confidentiality. Conversely many mental health services have joint agreements with statutory agencies regarding information sharing. This one issue has the potential in bringing working agreements to collapse if it is not explored and addressed in the early stages of any planned development for working within hospital and community settings.

There are inherent difficulties in working with dual diagnosis in homeless populations. Community substance misuse services provide community care assessments for detoxification and rehabilitation, however, there is no provision that has enabled funding dual diagnosis patients to specialist centres for treatment. Additionally, there is a distinct lack of inpatient detoxification and residential rehabilitation services for this client group. Whereas substance misuse patients can enter into rehabilitation which addresses their ability not only to remain drug free but offers rehabilitation into the wider community. This is not so with dual diagnosis patients and may result in inappropriate admissions to acute psychiatric services.

High levels of vulnerability are found in dual diagnosis populations, and when concerns are raised regarding mental health, many supervised hostels, mental health or substance misuse rehabilitation units state that they are not able to offer services to dual diagnosis patients. This is perhaps one of the most frustrating aspects of community dual diagnosis work. Concerns about mental health issues, psychopharmacology of mental health, dealing and drug and alcohol use on premises combined with a general housing shortage have often placed this client group outside any criteria established for different levels of housing or supported accommodation.

One of the most important considerations in community services for dual diagnosis is how all teams and services work together, collaboration and joint working practices can provide a comprehensive care package for dual diagnosis patients (Teague *et al.* 1995; Shwartz *et al.* 1997; Mueser *et al.* 1998). Many services developed both in the US, and more recently in the UK are based on a case management with the belief that this would reduce the number of crisis episodes and admissions (Shwartz *et al.* 1997). Breslow *et al.*'s (1996) study of an evaluation of the impact by managed care systems found that while managed care patients continued to require emergency services, patients who were not case managed required more interventions and showed more psychotic symptoms and substance use.

Professional development

One of the contentious topics in working with dual diagnosis is the need for appropriate staff training, support and supervision (Zweeben 1990; Siegfried *et al.* 1999; Sainsbury Centre 1999). It is essential that all staff have the opportunity to train in dual diagnosis. Cross training of mental health into addictions and addictions into mental health will enable nurses and other health care professionals who are already managing dual diagnosis patients to feel supported and raise competencies in clinical work areas. Additional education strategies for the individual with dual diagnosis are equally important, and must entail degrees of sophistication that enable service users to utilise and understand different programmes such as relapse prevention, and drug and alcohol education. A good background knowledge on the range of commonly misused substances including the physical and psychological effects will help the nurse to understand the nature of patients' symptoms. Therapeutic skills in assessment, motivational interviewing and relapse prevention, stress management, self-care activities and health education programmes) are important in identifying and helping those with a dual diagnosis to either abstain or moderate their use of substances (Gafoor & Rassool 1998). Educational systems that believe in providing information on substance misuse to psychiatric staff can enable more active care provision for this population (Ryrie & McGovan 1998; Siegfried *et al.* 1999).

Conclusion

Both addictions and psychiatry have well developed and established services, however, these services have developed different focuses for treatment. Substance misuse services encourage the patient to seek help, and see the individual as responsible for the actions and choices they make, psychiatry does not. Severe and enduring mental illness is often seen as the individual not being able to make safe choices, and at times not being responsible for their actions. These philosophies form the basis of treatment services, and in the case of psychiatry the ability to detain an individual under the Mental Health Act (1983) to ensure treatment. Within these frameworks, individuals who are seen as substance misusers with mental health problems were often seen as not wanting help, difficult to treat, unable to participate in counselling or psychotherapy due to the influence of psychoactive substances. Conversely, substance misuse services had difficulty in offering a service to individuals who have significant mental health problems and defaulted on addiction programme, or appointments. While both addiction and mental health services have dual diagnosis patients in treatment programmes, there are a significant number who fall between the service provisions due to the severity of their problems. This gives rise to the 'revolving door syndrome' for dual diagnosis patients who are seen as inappropriate to either service. Dual diagnosis services attempt to bridge this gap in the current service arrangements by addressing both the substance misuse and the mental health problems.

So, who is responsible for providing dual diagnosis services? All services have a role to play, whilst some may argue that specific services need to be established it is unlikely that separate funding of specific services will become available. Regardless of which agency takes a lead, nurses play a central role in the development of dual diagnosis practice, including designing and implementing a combined approach to working in dual diagnosis. Dual diagnosis cases are complex; one philosophy is that every agency has a role to play, and that we share the work equally. Individual case management works in parallel to nominated key worker CPA systems allowing for flexible working practices in all settings, including assertive outreach programmes which can be extended to joint working agreements with other agencies. The community responses to the health and social care needs of patients with mental health problems and substance misuse have, in the past, failed to provide adequate and accessible services. To some extent, this group has been marginalised by professionals and by society at large. Nurses work with dual diagnosis clients/patients every day, in all fields of nursing. As clinicians, nurses are ideally placed to both explore the issue of dual diagnosis in their own locality, or influence the ability for all services to work jointly on the issue of dual diagnosis.

References

Allen, K.M. & Gerace, L.M. (1996) Psychiatric nursing. In: K.M. Allen (ed.) *Nursing Care of the Addicted Client*. Lippincott, Philadelphia.

Breslow, R., Klinger, B. & Erickson, B. (1996) Characteristics of managed care patients in a psychiatric emergency service. *Psychiatric Services* **47** (11), 1259–1261.

Cabinet Office (1998) *Tackling Drugs to Build a Better Britain: The Government's 10-Year Strategy for Tackling Drug Misuse*, CM3945 9. The Stationery Office, London.

Carey, M.P., Carey, K.B. & Meisler, A.W. (1991) Psychiatric symptoms in mentally ill chemical abusers. *Journal of Nervous and Mental Diseases* **179**, 136–138.

Department of Health (1999) *National Service Framework for Mental Health*. The Stationery Office, London.

Department of Health (2000a) *Reforming the Mental Health Act*. The Stationery Office, London.

Department of Health (2000b) *Effective Care Co-Ordination in Mental Health Services: Modernising the Care Program Approach*, A Policy Booklet. The Stationery Office, London.

Dixon, L., Haas, J., Weiden, P., Sweeney, J. & Frances, A. (1990) Acute effects of drug abuse in schizophrenic patients: clinical observation and patients' self reports. *Schizophrenia Bulletin* **16** (1), 69–79.

Gafoor, M. (1985) Nurses attitudes to the drug abuser. Letter to *Nursing Times* 30 October.

Gafoor, M. (1997) Substance misuse and mental health. In: G. Hussein Rassool & M. Gafoor (eds) *Addiction Nursing — Perspectives on professional and clinical practice*. Stanley Thorne, Cheltenham.

Gafoor, M. & Rassool, G.H. (1998) The co-existence of psychiatric disorders and substance misuse: working with dual diagnosis patients. *Journal of Advanced Nursing* **27**, 497–502.

Greenman, D. (1994) The role of the addictions nurse specialist in adult psychiatry. *Perspectives on Addictions Nursing* **5** (3), 3–4.

McKeown, M. & Liebling, H. (1995) Staff perceptions of illicit drug use within a special hospital. *Journal of Psychiatric and Mental Health Nursing* **2** (6), 343–350.

Mueser, K.T., Bond, G.R., Drake, R.E. & Resnick, S.G. (1998) Models of community care for severe mental illness: A review of research on case management. *Schizophrenia Bulletin* **24**, 37–74.

Osher, F. & Kofoed, L. (1989) Treatment of patients with psychiatric and psychoactive substance abuse disorders. *Hospital and Community Psychiatry* **40** (10), 1025–1030.

Polcin, D. (1992) Issues in the treatment of dual diagnosis clients who have chronic mental illness. *Professional Psychology: Research and Practice* **23** (1), 30–37.

Rassool, G. Hussein (1993) Nursing and substance misuse: responding to the challenge. *Journal of Advanced Nursing* **18**, 1401–1407.

Rassool, G. Hussein (1997) Addiction nursing — towards a new paradigm: The UK experience. In: G. Hussein Rassool & M. Gafoor (eds) *Addiction Nursing — Perspectives on professional and clinical practice*. Stanley Thorne, Cheltenham.

Rassool, G. Hussein (1999) Addiction nursing: a community oriented approach. In: J. Littlewood (ed.) *Current Issues in Community Nursing*. Churchill Livingstone, Edinburgh.

Rassool, G. Hussein (2000) Addiction: global problem and global response, complacency or commitment? Editorial. *Journal of Advanced Nursing* **32** (3), 505–508.

Ryrie, I. & McGowan, J. (1998) Staff perceptions of substance use among acute psychiatry inpatients. *Journal of Psychiatric Mental Health Nursing* **5** (2), 137–142.

Scott, H., Johnson, S., Menzies, P. *et al.* (1999) Substance misuse and risk of aggression and offending among the severely mentally ill. *British Journal of Psychiatry* **172**, 345–350.

Shwartz, M., Baker, G., Mulvey, K. & Plough, A. (1997) Improving publicly funded substance abuse treatment: the value of case management. *American Journal of Public Health* **87** (10), 1659–1664.

Siegfried, N., Ferguson, J., Cleary, M., Walter, G. & Rey, J.M. (1999) Experience, knowledge and attitudes of mental health staff regarding patient' problematic drug and alcohol use. *Australian and New Zealand Journal of Psychiatry* **33** (2), 267–273.

Teague, G., Drake, R. & Ackerson, T. (1995) Evaluating the use of continuous treatment teams for persons with mental illness and substance abuse. *Psychiatric Services* **7**, 689–695.

Thacker, W. & Tremaine, L. (1989) Systems issues in serving the mentally ill substance abuser: Virginia's experience. *Hospital and Community Psychiatry* **40** (10), 1046–1049.

The Sainsbury Centre (1999) *Keys to Engagement*. London.

Tyrer, P., Coid, J., Simmonds, S., Joseph, P. & Marriot, S. (1997) Community mental health team management for those with severe mental illnesses and disordered personality. Cochrane Library, Oxford.

UKADCU (2000) *Pooled Treatment Budgets: Guidance to Drug Action Teams (2000)*. The UK Anti-Drugs Co-Ordination Unit, Cabinet Office, London.

Ward, M. & Applin, C. (1998) *The Unlearned Lesson. The Role of Alcohol and Drug Misuse in Homicides Perpetrated by People with Mental Health Problems*. Wynne Howard Books, Kenley.

Williams, R. (2000) Substance use and misuse in psychiatric wards. A model task for clinical governance? *Psychiatric Bulletin* **24**, 43–46.

Zweeben, J. (1993) Dual diagnosis: key issues for the 1990's. *Psychology of Addictive Behaviours* **7** (3), 168–172.

9: Enhancing the Social Service Response

Alison Keating

Introduction

The term dual diagnosis actually refers to the coexistence of any two medical diagnoses, but has come to be commonly associated with the concurrent existence of substance misuse and mental health problems. People with such a diagnosis are recognised as having complex needs, a term which reflects the wide variety of difficulties faced by this client group, many of which are social problems (Mind 1998); as such these clients can be regarded as doubly disadvantaged. As each problem is exacerbated by the other, these clients have much worse outcomes on most measures—housing status, employment status, social functioning and family relationships (Department of Health 1999a). It is increasingly being recognised that both health and social initiatives are necessary to deal with these clients (Ghodse *et al.* 1999). The literature on best practice with this client group is in its early stages, but evidence on the social work role in particular with comorbid clients is extremely limited.

Social workers work in a variety of settings with differing roles in purchasing and providing social work. Social workers located in specialist substance misuse teams or working within specialist mental health teams will have significant levels of intervention with clients who are dually diagnosed. Those placed within the homeless sector, children and families teams and acting as generic social workers for example, are likely to have less experience and cause to intervene with this group. Yet it is likely that all social workers have a valuable role to play in improving services for this group of clients. Information on prevalence will be considered elsewhere in this book, suffice to say 'given the extent of the problem, substance abuse among severely mentally ill patients should be considered usual rather than exceptional' (Smith & Hucker 1993). It is also recognised that among mentally disordered offenders, a client group in which social services will work, many will be dually diagnosed (Hudson *et al.* 1993) and use services more frequently (Department of Health 1999a). As there are factors associated with dual diagnosis such as poor medication compliance, higher susceptibility to high-risk behaviours, higher rates of hostility aggression and violence and increased rates of suicidal behaviour, it is apparent that many disciplines find this group difficult to manage. In their booklet *Understanding Dual Diagnosis*, Mind (1998) commented that this group '. . . have been regarded as difficult to treat, unresponsive and chaotic, and many workers feel unconfident in caring for such clients'. It is reasonable to suggest that this client group can feel alienated from services.

This chapter will consider the differing roles that social services have in relation to dually diagnosed clients and argues that a comprehensive and multifaceted approach in strategy development, commissioning and service provision is required to maximise the effectiveness of the social services' response. Components of the role of the specialist and non-specialist social worker are also considered. Appropriate training, which also has a valuable role in increasing confidence, is integral to such effective service provision and issues regarding training needs and provision are also explored.

Commissioning and strategy development

The current government (June 2001) has introduced a plethora of strategies, guidelines and frameworks for health and social services as part of its modernising agenda. The main thrust is the delivery of services in an effective, efficient and economic manner, developing partnerships and working collaboratively across sectors, increasing performance, utilising outcome measures, developing high quality services and the reduction of inequalities. In all aspects of provision services must elicit users' views and pay attention to the needs of carers. The importance of tackling substance misuse and mental health is integral to the government's agenda. The Cabinet paper concerning drugs, *Tackling Drugs to Build a Better Britain*, advises that services 'provide an integrated, effective and efficient response to people with drugs and mental health problems' (Cabinet Office 1998, p. 23). Specific mention is also made of substance misuse and mental health in the government's national priorities for health and social services. This includes expanding the capacity of substance misuse services, targeted prevention for young people most vulnerable to drug misuse and the development of assertive outreach teams for the mentally ill.

Modernising Mental Health Services—Safe, Sound and Supportive acknowledges the failure of care in the community. The document introduces National Service Frameworks to implement changes. The following principles underpin the frameworks, improved needs assessment, good risk management, early interventions, better outreach, additional beds and integrated forensic and secure provision. Additional funding is to be made available to meet these needs and responsibility for addressing the priority area of mental health is shared between social services and health. Given these strategic considerations social services will have a key role in contributing to the commissioning of effective services and should work towards increasing knowledge and information amongst social services staff as a whole. If social services departments are to enhance their role, consideration must also be given to wider environmental issues, promotion of economic regeneration, consideration of the effect of the built environment and contributing to strategies designed to target specific groups to name but a few. As a key department within local authorities, they should use their influence to ensure that the impact of initiatives on mental health and drugs is considered by all relevant departments.

Social services departments are in touch with many dually diagnosed clients and should consult widely with their clients and contribute fully to needs assessment. Consideration should be given to auditing practice within a variety of social services departments to assess and improve their own work and services with those vulnerable to substance misuse, e.g. in the field of housing and other agencies and services as regards factors ranging from recognition to service provision. Later in the chapter consideration will be given as to how social services can improve on these aspects of service provision.

The service provider role

Challenging attitudes

There are indications that some social workers can have very negative views with regard to substance misusers. 'Social workers negative attitudes to drinkers derive from feeling that they are inadequate to deal with alcohol problems, lack legitimacy and are unsupported by management' (Kent 1995). These feelings are likely to be enhanced when the client also presents with mental health problems. Both specialist and non-specialist social workers have a responsibility to attempt to identify and understand any negative feelings they may have about clients with substance use problems and recognise that various prejudices can be compounded. 'By definition, prejudiced attitudes and negative discrimination have no part in good practice' (Kent 1995).

As patients with mental health and substance misuse problems are often difficult to deal with there are likely to be negative stereotypes about this group and these may be exacerbated by other social stereotypes. It is recognised that it is the responsibility of all professionals to ensure that services for people who misuse alcohol and drugs are sensitive to needs associated with gender, race, culture, religion, language, employment status, parental or carer status, sexual orientation, lifestyle, HIV status, disability and age (SSI 1997), and social workers must consider how these factors may compound their negative attitudes to this client group. There is, for example, a general assumption that members of black and minority ethnic groups underutilise substance misusers services; however, in the mental health sector, black people represent a preponderance among service users. If substance misuse services are to be effective at attracting and retaining black and minority ethnic clients they must ensure that appropriate procedures are in place that recognise diversity and shared values and acknowledge the presence of institutional racism (McPherson 1999) which will affect their attitudes to black people with mental health problems who also misuse substances.

It is also recognised that the development of a non-judgemental relationship with a client can contribute to client motivation (Gafoor & Rassool 1997) and that all workers should discuss attitudes with a line manager or supervisor (Kent 1995). This means however, that social services managers need to be practised in tackling attitudes whilst being supportive and non-judgemental to their staff.

Specialist social workers

Most specialist social workers in substance misuse and/or mental health work within multidisciplinary teams. A number of models of working with dually diagnosed patients have emerged. Consecutive models involve treatment provided in a successive manner by the mental health services and substance misuse services depending on the presenting problem. Parallel treatment is when care is provided concurrently by both services, who communicate with one another or patients can be jointly managed by both services in an integrated fashion (Minkoff & Drake 1989; Franey & Quirk 1996). Some specialist dual diagnosis teams have been developed. Collaborative working is needed locally for social services and health to determine their model of service provision (Ghodse *et al.* 1999). In any case there is likely to be a need for training in either mental health or substance misuse for the specialist teams. Regardless of the model in which the practitioners are based, important components in the effective treatment of people with severe mental illness and substance misuse include: assertive outreach; close monitoring; supportive accommodation; careful timing of treatment interventions; taking a long-term therapeutic perspective and optimism factors (Drake *et al.* 1993).

Specialist social workers are likely to have the same needs as their colleagues in the multidisciplinary teams. The 1992 publication by CCETSW on competencies for social workers working with those with alcohol problems recognises that all post qualifying education and training programmes in this field are multidisciplinary. It is very important, therefore, that there are channels available for social workers to highlight their particular training needs.

Intensive case management

Specialist social workers should consider adopting an intensive case management model. Some American studies have indicated that enhanced social work services provided with drug treatment can lead to better outcomes. McLellan *et al.* (1998) undertook a controlled study, providing some drug treatment clients with social workers with additional budgets and access to community services. On virtually all of the outcome measures that they used, the group of patients who received enhanced services showed a better outcome. Fifty-five per cent of the group had received one specialised service from a professional in either the areas of medical or psychiatric care or a referral for housing or treatment. The logic underlying the study was that the social and medical needs of the client group impeded the progress of the clients and the 'addiction services combined with social services are the necessary conditions for truly effective treatment'. Although this study was undertaken with clients accessing drug treatment, many of the group were noted to have mental health problems and logic tells us that comorbid clients are even more likely to benefit from enhanced social work services. Drake *et al.* also states that there is evidence emerging from evaluation studies that these clients respond well to an assertive outreach approach and more intensive forms of case management, which will increase the client's retention in treatment and increase coping skills (Drake *et al.* 1993).

Assertive outreach is an important aspect of intensive case management and risk reduction and it is now government policy to develop these teams further. It is imperative that social services are fully involved in the extension of these teams. Their wide network of contacts needs to be amenable and supportive in contacting clients.

Social services managers are now involved in commissioning services jointly with health agencies for this group. They should ensure that they are fully briefed with all guidance, for commissioning standards developed by the Substance Misuse Advisory Services (HAS 2000) on issues of service specifications. In developing services consideration should also be given to the development of enhanced services. This would certainly complement the drive towards more assertive case management.

Care programme approach and risk management

The most appropriate tool in the provision of intensive care management for dually diagnosed clients is the Care Programme Approach (CPA). The Care Programme Approach was introduced in 1991 and updated in 1999. Its main requirement is that all patients referred to specialist psychiatric services have a systematic assessment of their health and social needs, a care programme that is appropriate to their needs and is agreed by care staff and family and a key worker allocated to monitor and review the patient's progress and continuing needs. The principles underpinning the CPA are the need for effective multidisciplinary and inter-agency working, ensuring users and carers are involved, assessing carers' needs and a recognition that the CPA details should be set at local levels (Department of Health 1995). *Building Bridges* (DoH 1995) was designed to advise on implementing the programme, and recognises the existence of dual diagnosis. It supports closer cooperation between the substance misuse and mental health services. But it is worth noting here that violence and criminal activity by clients should be considered as part of a comprehensive assessment.

125

Supervision registers were introduced to address the needs of people who are potentially at risk of harming themselves or others. Mentally ill patients considered at risk of committing serious violence, attempting suicide or severe self-neglect should be assessed as to whether they warrant inclusion on the supervision register. However, supervision registers are to be abolished in 2001 as a result of the need to ensure the provisions of services to the most vulnerable under the Care Programme Approach (Department of Health 1999e). Social workers in considering use of the Care Programme Approach should consider the views of Davies and Woolgrove (1998) in their review of the supervision register. They noted the impact of substance use on mental health and stated that the main problem was that as a non-statutory provision the register was being used inconsistently. They concluded that future developments depend on 'further improvements in the nature and quality of the working relationship between health and social care'. In relation to supervision orders Rorstad *et al.* (1996) commented that this power was not widely used with dually diagnosed patients and that consideration should be given as to how best to extend its use. It is hoped that these same criticisms cannot be made of the use of the CPA with this client group.

Thorough assessments are the key to providing a comprehensive and consistent approach to risk assessment and management and therefore contribute to protection of the individual and the wider community. The review of the Mental Health Act stressed the importance of not allowing substances to cloud assessments for mental illness. As such, the clear identification of dual disorders may only be achievable by observing patients over time (Franey & Quirk 1996). In this circumstance, the specialist social worker may need to work collaboratively with their generic colleagues to meet client need. They must also consider the entirety of services that should be involved in the assessment process. The National Service Frameworks have set standards that indicate that all mental health service users on CPA should receive care that optimises engagements, anticipates or prevents a crisis, and reduces risk. When appropriate, social workers should consider integrating CPA with their statutory responsibilities under the NHS and the Community Care Act and Mental Health Act. It reduces the number of assessment appointments and allows for one profession taking responsibility for coordinating all services. Integrated within into this process is the need for a full assessment of risk pertaining to the client themselves and colleagues. Managers should ensure that the care coordinator is able to combine the core coordinator and care management roles if integration of CPA and care management is to work (Department of Health 1999a).

In 1998 the Social Service Inspectorate (SSI) examined the arrangements for the integration of CPA and care management and found that local authorities had made progress in implementing the guidance (Department of Health 1999e). The process was updated in 1999 now providing for care coordinators rather than key workers, and moving toward joint training of health and social care staff, a common agreed risk assessment/management systems and a single point of access for assessments (Department of Health

1999d). It did state however, that many of the social services departments and NHS Trusts had difficulty agreeing management and budgetary arrangements through care management. The move toward joint commissioning should ease this process. It is important however, that the integration of CPA and social work statutory responsibilities is considered and that the service is extended to drug and alcohol services, many of whom do not routinely use the CPA at all.

Risk assessment and management within substance issue services is the key to the prevention of harm or negative consequences and reinforcing positive consequences in an environment of uncertainty (NHS Executive 1998). A good risk assessment policy with this client group will both reduce drug-related deaths, accidents and harm associated with substance misuse and protect individuals, their families, friends, carers and the community from drug-related harm (Cabinet Office 1998). All staff with the substance misuse services should receive training on risk assessment and management as part of induction to the service and ongoing personal and professional development (Department of Health 1999b). All social workers in contact with clients at risk of suicide should receive training in the recognition, assessment and management of risk, of both suicide and violence, at intervals of no more than three years (Department of Health 1999b). Undoubtedly this is not generally the case and departments and individual practitioners should take steps to ensure that the training needs of staff involved in this specialist area are investigated and addressed.

Specialist social workers undertaking community care assessments should ensure that these are client led and not determined purely by the resources available (Department of Health 1997; SSI 1997). The need for specialist community care assessors to have adequate training on substance misuse, mental health and the effect of one on the other is therefore evident. The Social Services Inspectorate makes specific mention of the need for assessment independent of providers. This would suggest that when community care assessors are placed within specialist teams, they need to take additional care to ensure that they are fully aware of all the options available to them. Operational goals ought to include attempting to create a systematic framework agreed across services and with service users with coordination as the key principle. This is ultimately compatible with developments in the move to a care-programming approach and problem-centred initiatives.

Non-specialist social workers

Recognition, prevention and early intervention

There are different issues to address when considering the role of generic and non-specialist social work staff with dually diagnosed clients: foremost amongst these is the issue of recognition. In 1978 Shaw *et al.* (1978) noted that practitioners often did not recognise the links between clients presenting problems and their pattern of alcohol consumption. Kent (1995) refers to anecdotal evidence that many social workers are aware of heavy drinking among the mentally ill, but are reluctant or afraid to become involved. Yet these clients are more likely to present themselves to helping agencies. This indicates the need for training and confidence building amongst this staff group.

If the drug prevention agenda is to be successful then there is an increased need for recognition, assessment and early intervention and it is important that social workers' networks and contacts with a variety of services and clients are utilised. For example social workers ought to discuss drinking patterns routinely in their contact with all clients and act appropriately on any information given. Lightfoot and Orford (1986) report a reluctance on the part of social workers to do so and that a lack of support from colleagues and supervisors exacerbates this reluctance. For example, people with complex drug and alcohol problems and severe mental illness are often found among the homeless population. Social workers working with the homeless are in a prime position to help these clients in accessing resources to increase their social stability. Non-specialist social workers will also need to be trained if they are to undertake effective assessments which consider the full complexity of a client's needs. 'Carrying out needs assessments on individuals which are not sensitive to the acceleration of problems brought about by layer upon layer of problems and triggering resources accordingly is short-termist and counterproductive' (Tickell 1999).

Social workers will also need to be fully involved with wider needs assessment in a locality and should be included on national and local database systems. In 1997, the SSI identified the possession of an information system that enables the department to record and evaluate the use made of services and to identify unmet need as an important performance indicator (SSI 1997). Additionally the current target led agenda would suggest the need for fully comprehensive baseline figures, which must incorporate social services information. It is of some concern that most social services departments do not return information to regional drugs misuse databases and many do not have local systems in place to record the totality of the department's contact with substance misusers.

Consideration will now be given to two specific aspects of the social work role and consideration given of how to address dually diagnosed clients within this context.

Child protection

Social work provision with children is governed by the Children Act (1989). One of the key principles of the Act is that the welfare of the child is the paramount consideration of a court; this represented a focus on child focused practice. Within this partnership with parents is encouraged, with parental care being the best for a child. Of most specific concern to those working within the drugs field is that the Act puts a duty on local authorities to safeguard and promote the welfare of the children within their area who are in need and to promote the upbringing of such children, by their families, by providing a range and level of services appropriate to each child's needs. This act also requires local authorities to prepare and assist those leaving the care of the local authority until they reach 21 years of age (Children Act 1989). Social workers in contact with dually diagnosed clients who also have children or young people with dual diagnosis who fit this criterion should ensure that they lobby for resources to meet the needs of this specialist group. Positive uses of the Children Act includes increased liaison with statutory services for the empowerment of clients (Kearney & Norman-Bruce 1993).

Many studies indicate the association of alcohol and drugs with child abuse (Mather 1988; Davidson 1992; Abel 1993). Mental health issues too are often a major factor in cases of child abuse. Practitioners need to be able to differentiate between managing a potentially harmful situation which may involve curtailing rights, for example access to small children at risk, and undertaking therapeutic work directed towards long-term behaviour change and rehabilitation (SCODA 1999). Many social workers may not be aware that the SSI has stated that having policy and procedures in place which clarify how child protection and mental health issues that arise in relation to substance misusers are dealt with is an important performance indicator. Conversely, substance misuse services should have childcare and child protection procedures (Kearney & Norman 1990). In order to ensure that children are protected, there is a need for social workers in children and families teams and those providing services to dually diagnosed clients to share skills and work collaboratively.

Young people

Prevention of substance misuse problems and mental health is very much part of the current agenda. The SCODA and Children's Legal Centre (1999) amongst others suggest that there are specific groups of vulnerable young people who may benefit from targeted early drug prevention approaches. Much the same group is vulnerable to mental health difficulties. These include:

- Those looked after or supervised by local authorities.
- Those excluded or disaffected from schools.
- Those who are homeless or local authority care leavers.
- Those living in difficult family circumstances.
- Those with drug or alcohol misusing parents.
- Those with physical disabilities and learning difficulties.

All of the above groups are likely to have contact with social services. Zeitlin (1999) suggests that the heterogeneity of young people with comorbidity for psychiatric disorder and substance misuse suggests that some would be better considered children with multiple problems, for whom the necessary conditions are vulnerability, lack of family protection and exposure to a source of drugs. He states that children who present with comorbidity are at very high risk. Reduction of this risk can be achieved by early identification and treatment of the comorbid condition and vigilance for substance misuse in all cases. Social services are the key to meeting the needs of young people vulnerable to physical and psychiatric disorder and ensuring the coordination of efforts from health, social services and education.

When providing treatment to young people, services should ensure that all interventions are undertaken in accordance with the guiding principle of the Children Act (1989): that the welfare of the child is paramount. The practitioner should adhere to local policies and procedures that are agreed with the relevant Area Child Protection Committee. It is important to consider the wider environment, to be comprehensive and to involve parents. Services should be able to provide long-term follow-up, where appropriate. Smith (2000), when referring to early intervention programmes with children affected by drugs, commented that whilst early intervention programmes may have a time-limited impact without continued support, pervasive social problems and poverty for example may counteract many of the early gains achieved in these programmes. One of the clear duties placed on social services is the protection of children and young people and they must be the key partners in meeting the needs of vulnerable young people.

Training

The earlier review of social work involvement with dually diagnosed clients points to the need for training to be given to social workers. Whilst there is evidently the need for appropriately informed and skilled interventions delivered by knowledgeable practitioners, there is ample scope for the application of more generalised knowledge and skills in this field. Central to avoiding such problems is the demystification of drugs and drug-related issues, so that mental health practitioners are enabled and empowered to practise skills that they already possess with the relevant client group (Derricott & Mckeown 1996). On the topic of substance misuse, CCETSW has pointed out that the call for such training from the social workers themselves is likely to be low (Kent 1995), particularly given the issues of confidence and attitudes highlighted previously. Social services departments should take steps to actively encourage staff participation in training around this issue.

Any systematic approach to meeting staff training needs should acknowledge and build upon existing competencies as a first step (Derricott & Mckeown 1996). If effective joint working is to take place it will also be important to learn about the roles of other agencies and the parameters of their interventions. In other spheres it has been recognised that the issues raised by individuals can be the basis of learning and that mutual learning can strengthen links between the social work and psychiatric professions. (CCETSW 1992). Any local training initiatives should ensure that social work needs are addressed and that there are avenues for practitioners to declare their training needs. Continued support must however, be provided whilst in the workplace if training is to be effective. Such supervision may need to be provided by a non-social worker, if the social worker's line manager is not experienced in working in this field (Kent 1995). Whilst Kent was referring to work with alcohol misusers this is true across the spectrum.

Issues that could usefully be covered in training for managers, purchasers and practitioners include:
• Attitudes to drug users — developing a non-judgemental attitude.
• Awareness of the effects and health risks of different drugs and assessment of substance use.
• Awareness of the interactions between substance misuse and mental health.
• Basic health care needs of substance misusers.
• Brief interventions and motivational interviewing.
• Child protection.
• Appropriate after care and community support.
• Mental health issues (including suicide and risk assessment).
• Service provision, targeting referrals and liaison (substance misuse and mental health).
• Basic health care needs of substance misusers.
• Substance misuse interventions and outcomes.
The training chosen will be dependent on the background and knowledge of the individual to be trained.

Conclusion

Social services departments have a key role in providing effective and efficient services to dually diagnosed patients. Many documents have referred to the need for improved liaison between Community Mental Health Teams, Community Drug and Alcohol Teams and primary care services (Department of Health 1999a). The need to involve social workers fully is also recognised in this country (Department of Health 1999a). The government's current strategy of joint management aims to increase the opportunity for skills sharing across agencies. The social services response needs to be wide-ranging and include effective and efficient arrangements for joint working and coordination of prevention, care and treatment and support for independence in the community by this client group (SSI 1997).

Non-specialist social workers should be trained in order to build up their confidence in working with this client group and in order to form part of a network of services that reach out to the dually diagnosed. Specialist social workers could consider their role in intensive case management. Case management has been described as a 'co-ordinated approach to the delivery of health, substance abuse, mental health, and social services, linking clients with appropriate services to address specific needs and achieve stated goals' (Siegal, 1998). Evidence indicates that a case management approach leads to better retention and better outcomes as it focuses on the whole individual and stresses comprehensive assessment, service planning and service coordination to address multiple aspects of a client's life.

All the evidence therefore points to the need to provide intensive care management with social services utilising its contacts and resources to enhance the efficacy of working together. If this is undertaken, then risks would be reduced and treatment effectiveness maximised.

References

Abel, C. (1993) *Child Abuse and Neglect: The Role of Protective Services*. University of Iowa, Iowa City.

Cabinet Office (1998) *Tackling Drugs to Build a Better Britain: the Government's 10-Year Strategy for Tackling Drug Misuse*, Cm 3945 9. The Stationery Office, London.

Central Council for Education and Training in Social Work and Royal College of Psychiatrists Symposium (1992) A Double Challenge—Working with people who have both learning difficulties and a mental illness. CCETSW.

Children Act (1989) HMSO, London.

Davidson, G. (1992) Problem Drinking as a Factor in Cases of Child Mistreatment—Comments and Observations. Alcohol Concern, Wales, unpublished report.

Davies, M. & Woolgrove, M. (1998) Mental health social work and the use of supervision registers for patients at risk. *Health and Social Care in the Community* **6** (1), 25–34.

Department of Health (1995) *Building Bridges—a Guide to Arrangements for Inter-Agency Working for the Care and Protection of Severely Mentally Ill People*. The Stationery Office, London.

Department of Health (1997) Purchasing effective treatment and care for drug misusers. *Guidance for Health Authorities and Social Services Department*. Department of Health, London.

Department of Health (1999a) Effective care co-ordination in mental health services. *Modernising the Care Programme Approach—a Policy Document*. Department of Health, London.

Department of Health (1999b) *Expert Seminar on Dual Diagnosis and Management of Complex Needs*. Department of Health, London.

Department of Health (1999c) Safer services. *National Inquiry into Suicide and Homicide by People with Mental Illness*. Department of Health, London.

Department of Health (1999d) *National Service Framework for Mental Health: Modern Standards & Service Models*. Department of Health, London.

Department of Health (1999e) *Still Building Bridges: The report of a national inspection of arrangements for the integration of care programme approach with care management*. Department of Health, London.

Derricott, J. & Mckeown, M. (1996) Dual diagnosis: future directions in training. *Association of Nurses in Substance Abuse Journal, Psychiatric Care* **12** (Suppl. 1), London.

Drake, R.E., Bartels, S.J., Teague, G.B., Noordsy, D.L. & Clark, R.E. (1993) Treatment of substance abuse in severely mentally ill patients. *Journal of Nervous and Mental Disease* **181**, 606–611.

Franey, C. & Quirk, A. (1996) *Dual Diagnosis, Executive Summary Number 51*. The Centre for Research on Drugs and Health Behaviour, London.

Gafoor, M. & Rassool, G. Hussein (1997) The co-existence of psychiatric disorders and substance misuse: working with dual diagnosis patients. *Journal of Advanced Nursing* **27**, 497–502.

Ghodse, A.H., Oyefeso, A., Clancy, C. et al. (1999) *Assessing the Need for a Dual Diagnosis Service for Substance Misusers and Mental Health Clients Using Programmatic Data in Haringey Healthcare NHS Trust*. Centre for Addiction Studies, St George's Hospital Medical School, London.

HAS (2000) *Commissioning Standards Drug and Alcohol Treatment and Care*. The Substance Misuse Advisory Service, London.

Hudson, B., Cullen, R. & Roberts, C. (1993) *Training for Work with Mentally Disordered Offenders. Report of a Study of the Training Needs of Probation Officers and Social Workers*. CCETSW, London.

Kearney, P. & Norman, B.G. (1990) Who's minding the kids. *Drug Link*, Vol. 5, No. 5.

Kearney, P. & Norman-Bruce, G. (1993) The Children Act. *Druglink* January/February.

Kent, R. (1995) *Alcohol Interventions: Guidelines for Social Workers, Employers and Training Programmes*. CCETSW, London.

Lightfoot, P. & Orford, J. (1986) 'Helping agents' — attitudes towards alcohol-related problems: situations vacant? *British Journal of Addiction* **81**, 749–756.

Mather, B. (1988) Child mistreatment and the misuse of alcohol. Occasional paper, Social Services Department, Devon County Council, Exeter.

McLellan, A.T., Hagan, T.A., Levine, M. *et al.* (1998) Supplemental social services improve outcomes in public addiction treatment. *Addiction* **93** (10), 1489–1499.

McPherson, W. (1999) *Stephen Lawrence. Report of an Inquiry*, Cm 4262–1. The Stationery Office, London.

Mind (1998) *Understanding Dual Diagnosis*. Mind, London.

Minkoff, K. & Drake, R.E.(1989) An integrated treatment model for dual diagnosis of psychosis and addition. *Hospital and Community Psychiatry* **40**, 10.

NHS Executive (1998) Management of uncertainty and communication of risk by clinicians. http://www.doh.gov.uk/ntrd/rd/implem/priority/first/03.htm. SCODA and Children's Legal Centre, London.

Rorstad, P., Checinski, K., McGeachy, O. & Ward, M. (1996) *Dual Diagnosis: Facing the Challenge*. Wynne Howard Publishing, Kenley.

Scoda and the Children's Legal Centre (1999) *Young people and drugs: Policy guidance for drug interventions*. Scoda & the Children's Legal Centre, London.

Shaw, S., Cartwright, A., Striptey, T. & Harwin, J. (1978) *Responding to Drinking Problems*. Croom Helm, London.

Siegal, H.A. (1998) *Comprehensive Case Management for Substance Abuse Treatment; Treatment Improvement Protocol (TIP)* Series 27. US Department of Health and Human Services, Public Health Service, Substance Abuse and Mental Health Administration, Centre for Substance Abuse Treatment. Rockville. MP 20857.

Smith, I. (2000) The Ecological Perspective: The impact of culture and social environment on drug-exposed children; in identifying the needs of drug affected children: public policy issues. OSAP Prevention Monograph — 11. US Department of Health and Human Services, Washington DC.

Smith, J. & Hucker, S. (1993) Dual diagnosis patients: substance abuse by the severely mentally ill. *British Journal of Hospital Medicine* **50** (1), 650–654.

Social Services Inspectorate (1997) *Inspection of Social Services for People who Misuse Alcohol and Drugs: Standards and Criteria*. Department of Health, London.

Tickell, C. (1999) Co-morbidity — the social implications. *Drugs: Education, Prevention and Policy* **6** (2), 175–179.

Zeitlin, H. (1999) Psychiatric co-morbidity with substance misuse in children and teenagers. *Drug and Alcohol Dependence* **55** (3), 225–234.

10: Treatment Strategies and Interventions

Ken Checinski

Introduction

Dual diagnosis presents one of the greatest challenges to mental health and substance misuse treatment agencies (Rorstad & Checinski 1996). This is not merely because of the extent of the problem, but also because it provokes us to think about how services work together. In England and Wales, the Care Programme Approach (NHS Management Executive 1994) was developed in response to a number of tragic incidents, that, when reviewed, showed some deficiencies in communication and collaboration between health and social care agencies in particular. Hitherto, there has been little encouragement for services to work together, apart from a pragmatic realisation that failure to do so can lead to futile interventions that are destined to failure, or, occasionally, even more unfortunate consequences for the individual concerned and, rarely, for society at large. This situation emphasises importance of a holistic, bio-psychosocial approach.

Diagnostic issues

Following something of an antipsychiatry backlash and its consequences in the 1970s and 1980s, the issue of 'diagnosis' has become more important and acceptable at various levels again. Interestingly, non-medical disciplines and non-health care agencies now talk enthusiastically about 'dual diagnosis', sometimes having been equally scathing about (single) diagnosis as a concept and a practice. The term 'complex needs' has been coined, in part to address the issues surrounding this paradox. Therefore, 'dual diagnosis' should be seen as a generic index of complexity as well as a diagnostic entity. It is becoming a 'ticket of entry' to services where needs-based targeting is increasingly applied to the allocation of resources where demand far outstrips supply. Diagnosis is more difficult because of the range of conditions involved. For example, if there are 12 broad diagnostic categories encountered by mental health services and 8 broad categories of substance misuse seen by drug and alcohol services, then a dual diagnosis approach must respond to 96 permutations. Even if dual diagnosis focuses on 'pure' schizophrenia or 'pure' manic-depressive illness, ignoring the importance of personality and neurotic disorders, there are still 16 permutations.

Diagnostic uncertainty is another confounding factor. Misdiagnosis occurs more frequently (Cohen 1995). Many patients with a dual diagnosis label have been given multiple diagnoses previously. If a certainty of 80% is assumed for each category of diagnosis, then the resulting dual probability is 64% (80%×80%), a poor starting point for planning a sophisticated care package. Then, many patients appear to merit a third diagnosis along the axis of personality disorder, which may have an even lower certainty still of about 60%. This gives a diagnostic precision of 38% for the most difficult cases. The figures suggested are open to question and reflect practice in the field rather than research precision. There is 'contamination' between diagnostic categories, with, for instance, borderline personality disorder including substance misuse as a criterion, while a significant number of substance misusers have 'borderline' features such as impulsivity and self-harm as part of their range of maladaptive coping behaviours.

Diagnostic drift and shift can also undermine treatment. Most significant mental health problems and much problematic substance misuse are chronic conditions. As time passes, with repeated treatment 'failures', patients may show diagnostic drift in an attempt to explain the poor outcome. Typically, patients may acquire a diagnosis of personality disorder, which has a poor prognosis. Hitherto, services have tended to see such patients as untreatable. Now, though, there is increased expectation that they are treated, as least in crisis, because of appropriate concern about suicides and homicides by 'mentally ill' patients in the community. Paradoxically, single diagnosis patients often have a chronic course: psychotic illnesses such as schizophrenia and manic depression are, by definition, long term, and drug and alcohol dependence syndromes are characterised by their relapsing, remitting nature. Why dual diagnosis should have a better prognosis, and therefore respond to well circumscribed intervention, is not entirely clear. Whilst drift occurs over a period of time, diagnostic shift may happen suddenly, usually in crisis, when there may be a decision to redefine the 'primary' diagnosis, thus assigning responsibility to either substance misuse or mental health teams, perhaps arbitrarily.

Diagnostic hierarchy also causes confusion (Rorstad & Checinski 1996). Traditionally, conditions higher up the diagnostic pyramid are seen as being able to cause features suggestive of disorders lower down:

- organic brain disease
- psychotic illness
- neurotic illness
- personality disorder
- behavioural problems.

For example, a brain tumour (organic brain disease) can produce symptoms and signs mimicking schizophrenia (psychotic illness); and psychotic illness can mimic personality disorder. Substance misuse does fit easily into this scheme, probably having causes and effects at all five levels. The hierarchical model is useful, but it can lead to misunderstanding, even in general mental health care. For instance, depression is a common feature in schizophrenia and can respond to changes in antipsychotic medication and to psychosocial interventions, rather than assuming that specific treatment for depressive disorder is required, such as antidepressant medication. Of course, multiple diagnoses can occur even within this hierarchy and should be treated appropriately. Terminology is confusing. Depression as a symptom is so common as to be almost normal (Checinski 1998). It is often used in place of the term depressive disorder or illness. The latter implies utilising a range of specific interventions (including medication, psychological treatments and social manipulation); the former should be an entrée to further diagnostic enquiry. Similarly, the term 'psychosis' is used very imprecisely, sometimes indicating psychiatric illnesses such as schizophrenia or manic depression, and sometimes merely implying a psychological detachment from reality (such as might occur with intoxication or borderline personality disorder).

Diagnostic precision is affected by the level of training of the professional concerned. Increasingly, since the early 1980s, mental health care and substance misuse treatment are being delivered by multidisciplinary teams. This is entirely appropriate, but raises the question of who makes the diagnosis. General practitioners refer some, but not all, patients to mental health services. Many substance misuse services encourage self-referral. Many patients coming to either service are not seen by a senior psychiatrist for a full assessment, but by someone who often has to rely on opinions from other, experienced colleagues in other disciplines. However, these disciplines are not trained to make diagnostic decisions. In fact, much non-medical training has been influenced by an active or passive antipsychiatry shift, such that many basic, professional training schemes place less emphasis on the particular place of diagnosis than in the past. Also, very few basic professional courses place much emphasis on substance misuse issues, despite their substantial influence on general health, mental health and social well-being. Even senior general adult psychiatrists may not be trained and up-to-date in dual diagnosis, given the small number of suitable substance misuse training opportunities available to them in the past, where it has been regarded as Cinderella psychiatry's disadvantaged sibling. Substance misuse services may be even more poorly equipped to make robust diagnoses, especially if they are provided by agencies with limited psychiatric input, perhaps a sessional general practitioner or even no medical input at all. Substance misuse teams appropriately draw staff from a range of backgrounds, including ex-misusers. However, unless there is diagnostic support and supervision, and orientation to the issues, they are poorly prepared to negotiate care packages with mental health teams for patients with dual diagnosis.

Disadvantage and outcome expectation

Poor prognosis and low expectation are reinforced by additional disadvantages, accentuated by the presence of both substance misuse and mental disorder, for example:

(1) Supported housing is in short supply for people with both mental health problems and substance misuse. This leads to the lack of a secure base for the individual and the lack of an anchor for services often tied to catchment areas or general practice lists. This exacerbates difficulties in communication and collaboration.

(2) There is usually significant educational disadvantage. Drug misuse and some mental disorders (especially schizophrenia and personality disorders) often have their roots in adolescence: this interferes with educational attainment and vocational training.

(3) Financial disadvantage is usual because of decreased capacity for work. Work is often menial, poorly paid and punctuated by relapses.

(4) Family life is adversely affected. Upbringing may be stormy, current support poor and relationships relatively chaotic. In addition, there may be justifiable concerns about childcare ability.

(5) General health is frequently poor, being affected by poverty and social marginalisation, as well as by the direct consequences of substance misuse. Patients may use primary health care, including screening programmes, poorly, often accessing their primary care in emergencies only through accident and emergency departments. Many general practitioners feel poorly placed to offer treatment for substance misuse, preferring to send patients to specialist services which may have long waiting lists for treatment.

Recurrent treatment failure may result in blame being placed on any or all the parties involved (patient, mental health team, substance misuse team, and other agencies). This can lead to frustration, misunderstanding and anger which can then cause further miscommunication, poor collaboration and therapeutic pessimism, ultimately increasing the chances of mismanagement of the case.

Intervention strategies for care and treatment

It is important to distinguish clinical treatment from general care, which includes housing, financial, educational, and vocational intervention. General health care should not be forgotten. Clinical treatment can be described as processes and primary responsibilities, and be qualified by possible pitfalls. Drake *et al.* (1993) and Johnson (1997) examine some of the pitfalls in more detail. Good practice in multidisciplinary assessment is described by Ghodse (1995). Table 10.1 summarises the issues already identified. The list of possible pitfalls suggests appropriate proactive and remedial action at several levels.

Most importantly, the knowledge, skills and attitudes of individual team members should be updated to address dual diagnosis issues, and due attention should be paid to recognising perceived and actual philosophical differences between mental health and substance misuse services.

Recognition should be given to the extra time required to assess and treat

Table 10.1 Clinical treatment

Process	Primary responsibility	Possible pitfalls
Screening	Any discipline	Training deficiency Attitudinal bias Lack of time Misleading clinical state
Brief intervention	Any discipline	Poor outcome caused by unrecognised complex problems
Diagnostic assessment	Psychiatrist or other appropriate doctor supported by other disciplines	Training deficiency Attitudinal bias, including perceived or actual philosophical differences
Review of diagnosis	Any clinical discipline, supported by psychiatrist or other appropriate doctor	Training deficiency Lack of time Misleading clinical state Failure to resolve diagnostic disagreement
Single team treatment	Either mental health team or substance misuse team	Skills deficiency Failure to agree fully that only one team should be involved Failure to target problem (does not meet criteria for single service) Lack of support (perceived or actual) for emergent diagnostic or therapeutic issues from the complementary team, leading to failure to involve that team
Dual team treatment	Mental health team and substance misuse team	Inappropriate (team or discipline) key worker allocation Communication problems related either to poor structures (meetings, clinical notes/correspondence) or mismatched policies and procedures Difficulty agreeing appropriate outcomes (e.g. abstinence from substances, stability of mental state) Failure to agree contingencies and boundaries (e.g. criteria for emergency intervention, including admission) Failure to communicate contingencies and boundaries to other professionals (e.g. out-of-hours services) Failure to resolve difficulties Sterile arguments about 'primary' problems within a fluid clinical picture Lack of appropriate assessment and treatment facilities (assessment beds, day hospital, etc.)

dual diagnosis patients. This means that, within finite resources, other patients will receive less input because of re-targeting. For example, detoxification should be supplemented by a period of time assessing the drug- and alcohol-free mental state; and patients with mental health problems should more frequently have biochemical testing for substance misuse.

Disagreement within teams and between teams about diagnosis, treatment and division of labour must be resolved.

Targeting criteria should allow for the complexity and needs presented by dual diagnosis, and policies and procedures for information sharing across teams and agencies (including confidentiality) should be designed to promote joint treatment where necessary.

Appropriate expectations and clinical outcomes should be agreed to minimise treatment 'failure' and therapeutic pessimism.

Contingencies and boundaries (including default options) should be agreed prior to treatment to avoid confusion and to prevent patients 'falling through the net'.

Communication channels, both informal and formal (e.g. use of the Care Programme Approach), should be open and designed to address disagreement, rather than ignore or perpetuate it.

All disciplines should appreciate the difficulty in identifying a 'primary' diagnosis (especially in crisis) and design treatment plans accordingly.

Table 10.2 summarises the care issues. Possible pitfalls suggest appropriate action at a number of levels within several teams and agencies:

- Specialist housing provision should be encouraged for people with dual diagnosis by ensuring appropriate support is available, including suitable funding levels, where enhanced staffing is needed.
- Specialist rehabilitation facilities and networks should become more oriented to the needs of patients with dual diagnosis. This will involve improvements in knowledge and skills and, sometimes, significant attitudinal changes.
- Concerns about education should be addressed and all round low expectations challenged constructively.
- Vocational services should become more oriented to the needs of patients with dual diagnosis. Low expectations should be addressed.
- Financial disadvantage should be addressed by tackling unrealistic expectations and by offering advice and training on budgeting, where necessary.
- Family interventions should be used where there are high levels of conflict or over-involvement, a history of family problems such as sexual abuse, or childcare issues. Child protection must be treated as a priority, both openly and fairly.
- Primary health care teams should be encouraged to deliver all facets of good general health care (e.g. screening and early intervention) by providing support and training, where appropriate.

Table 10.2 Care issues

Process	Primary responsibility	Possible pitfalls
Housing provision	Local authority Social services Housing associations Rehabilitation networks	Housing provision focused on substance misuse or mental health problems, not tolerant of, or familiar with, the complementary problems, leading to rapid breakdown of placement Perceived or actual lack of support from appropriate teams Rehabilitation provision and support not equipped to deal with dual diagnosis Funding disagreements where budgets are separate
Educational disadvantage	Local authority	Adult learning may be seen as threatening or financially unappealing by patient Low value placed on remedial education by patient Low expectation by teams
Vocational disadvantage	Vocational training services	Vocational training may be seen as threatening or financially unappealing by patient Low value placed on work by patient Low expectation by teams
Financial disadvantage	Social services Department of Social Services	Perceived and actual prioritisation of spending on substance misuse by patient Patient has poor budgeting skills
Family problems	Any discipline Child and family services	Difficulty engaging sometimes chaotic families Actual and perceived threat to patient because of childcare issues
General health	Any discipline Primary health care teams	Training deficiency Attitudinal bias Primary heath care team members feel de-skilled when treating these patients
	Effects of chronic poor	Health

Specific therapeutic interventions

Therapeutic interventions should be based on a bio-psychosocial paradigm. These three domains overlap to a certain extent. For example, certain depressive disorders respond equally well to cognitive behaviour therapy or antidepressant medication.

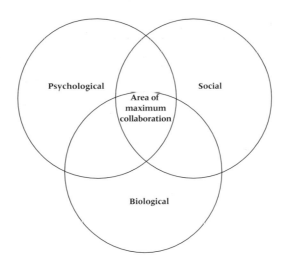

Fig. 10.1 Domains for
therapeutic intervention

Figure 10.1 illustrates the need for effective collaboration between disciplines and teams, showing the greatest overlap as the 'area of maximum collaboration'. It is difficult to envisage how all the necessary interventions, including those designed to meet care issues, could be consistently met within a single team, which would have to be so big as to be unwieldy. Dedicated dual diagnosis teams are described but have not become widespread (Drake *et al.* 1993; Galanter *et al.* 1994). They may be perceived as too expensive and too highly specialised to address such a broad range of issues. Ley *et al.* (2000) summarise three permutations of approach:

(1) *Serial*: psychiatric and substance misuse treatments occur in sequence (either comes first, depending on clinical state).

(2) *Parallel*: concurrent but separate psychiatric and substance misuse treatment.

(3) *Integrated*: concurrent treatment by a single team.

Liaison and care brokerage models are popular but evidence for their effectiveness is minimal (Weaver *et al.* 1999). Assertive community teams are of unproven benefit to patients with dual diagnosis. The choice of model will depend on current service structures. Strong community services may be more likely to benefit from a liaison approach, while either an assertive community approach or a dedicated team is viable where there is higher population density, such as in urban settings. Whatever model is chosen, many patients will not fit neatly into it. Therefore, it is important to have a strong key worker system to enable effective brokerage of the network of treatment and care required. This can be conceptualised as a 'virtual' team, having the advantage of flexibility, but lacking the cohesion of a single 'physical' team.

Figure 10.2 shows some of the components of a 'virtual' team approach, redefining the patient and key worker as the 'focus for maximum collaboration'.

141

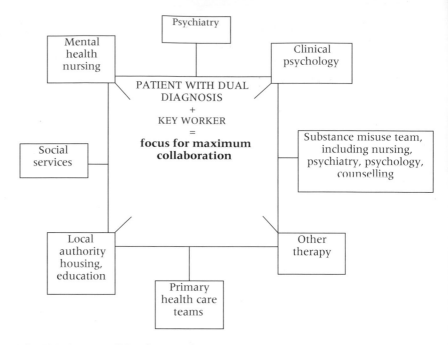

Fig. 10.2 Conceptualising the 'virtual team'

Biological interventions

Detoxification

If a patient is physically dependent on alcohol, opioids (e.g. heroin or methadone), or sedative-hypnotics (e.g. diazepam, barbiturates), detoxification is required to prevent withdrawal effects and complications. There is no significant physical dependence on stimulants, hallucinogens, cannabis or solvents. During any form of detoxification, special attention must be paid to assessing changes in the mental state, including risk factors for accidental or deliberate self-harm. Patients with dual diagnosis should be considered for inpatient treatment if a community approach is inadequate. .

Alcohol detoxification using diazepam

This should be a short course. Poor compliance and risk of overdose may necessitate inpatient treatment.

A typical specimen regime might be as follows:

Diazepam 10 mg qds for 1 day

10 mg tds for 1 day

5 mg qds for 1 day

5 mg tds for 1 day

5 mg bd for 1 day

5 mg nocte for 1 day

Start at 15 mg qds if there have been severe withdrawal states in the past.

Avoid oral chlormethiazole because of the toxic interaction with alcohol (McInnes 1987): this is especially important for community detoxification. If there is concurrent benzodiazepine misuse, the doses and length of treatment may require slight augmentation.

Opioid detoxification using methadone

This requires stabilisation on an appropriate dose of oral methadone and dose reduction over 2–4 weeks. This is suitable for patients with a short history of opioid dependence and/or a high level of motivation.

Opioid detoxification using a partial agonist

This is usually carried out with a medication such as sublingual buprenorphine. This is safer in overdose than methadone but is potentially injectable and harder to supervise.

Opioid detoxification is also performed with other oral medications such as dihydrocodeine but this is potentially injectable and has no advantages over standard detoxification using oral methadone.

Opioid detoxification giving symptomatic relief only

A typical specimen regime for this intervention might be as follows:
Thioridazine 25 mg bd and 50–100 mg nocte for 7–10 days, and
Diphenoxylate hydrochloride (Lomotil) 2 tablets qds for 3 days
2 tablets tds for 2 days
2 tablets bd for 2 days
Clonidine (an α_2-agonist) can be used, although there may be problems of hypotension during treatment and rebound hypertension on discontinuation. Lofexidine has a central action like clonidine, but is less likely to cause hypotension. A specimen regime for lofexidine is as follows.
Initially 200–400 mg bd, then increase in 200–400 mg steps to 2.4 g per day, depending on the presence or absence of objective withdrawal symptoms and signs
Administer for 7–10 days, then taper off over 2–4 days (watch for rebound hypertension).

Benzodiazepine detoxification for sedative–hypnotic dependence (including barbiturates)

It is important to substitute a long-acting benzodiazepine and then reduce the dose gradually with support and advice about rebound anxiety and insomnia. For example, it would be necessary for a patient to change from lorazepam to diazepam. The length of detoxification depends on the severity and chronicity of the dependence. Barbiturate withdrawal may be done using reducing doses of a barbiturate such as phenobarbitone.

Chronic opioid dependence may be alleviated by longer term prescription of methadone in association with a comprehensive range of psychosocial interventions. The term 'methadone maintenance' refers to higher dose methadone (80–120 mg daily) given as a part of a comprehensive care plan designed to lead to psychosocial stability and subsequent detoxification.

Relapse prevention

Opioid dependence

Naltrexone can be started 7–10 days after detoxification and given three times a week because of its long half-life. It blocks the effects of opioid drugs. It can cause hepatotoxicity, so liver function should be monitored.

Alcohol dependence

Naltrexone may reduce reinstatement of drinking by reducing craving and abolishing the initial euphoriant effect (O'Malley *et al.* 1992; Volpicelli *et al.* 1992). Acamprosate (a synthetic gamma-amino butyric acid (GABA) analogue) has a similar effect (Lhuitre *et al.* 1990). Disulfiram (Antabuse) inhibits the aldehyde dehydrogenase acetaldehyde reaction. Daily compliance is a problem: supervision is likely to increase both compliance and the chances of alcohol abstinence (Heather *et al.* 1993). Unsupervised disulfiram is not very fruitful (Fuller *et al.* 1986) — nor are implants (Morland *et al.* 1984).

Psychological interventions

Insight-oriented psychotherapy is suitable for patients with good motivation who, nevertheless, have entrenched regressive and self-destructive thoughts and impulses. Psychotherapeutic techniques are widely used in many forms of mental health disorder and substance misuse problem (Kaufman 1994). Counselling approaches are also used specifically in dual diagnosis cases (Evans & Sullivan 1990).

Behavioural psychotherapy can help to abolish learned responses. Cue exposure has been shown to extinguish responses to acquired drinking cues (Glautier & Drummond 1994).

Motivational interviewing is a cognitive behavioural technique that proposes that there are both costs and benefits of substance misuse to the individual (Miller 1983). It allows the development and consolidation of the need to change by using several techniques (Miller & Rollnick 1991):
- deliberate expression of empathy;
- avoiding arguments;
- detection of, and 'rolling' with, resistance;
- highlighting discrepancies in the patient's history; and
- drawing out the patient's discomfort about the substance misuse.

Interestingly, motivational interviewing has been adapted to increase the compliance with treatment of acutely psychotic patients (Kemp *et al.* 1996).

Cognitive psychotherapy, using the model of relapse (Marlatt & Gordon 1985), is a mainstay of relapse prevention. It has a number of key features:

- recognising exposure to high risk situations;
- using coping responses for high risk situations;
- distinguishing between lapse and relapse;
- acquiring self-efficacy; and
- developing a healthier lifestyle.

Approaches such as controlled drinking may be used, involving structured self-control training (Heather & Robertson 1983).

Self-directed and brief therapies have several key features:

- Low cost.
- Involve modest time investment.
- Promote self-help and self-management.
- Have minimal professional involvement.

Structure is important: using a self-help manual is better than minimal advice alone (Heather *et al.* 1986).

The acronym 'FRAMES' summarises the elements of effective brief interventions (Bien *et al.* 1993):

F: *FEEDBACK* of personal risk or impairment
R: emphasis on personal *RESPONSIBILITY* for change
A: clear *ADVICE* to change
M: a *MENU* of alternative change options
E: therapeutic *EMPATHY* as a counselling style
S: enhancement of patient *SELF-EFFICACY* or optimism
Follow-up enhances maintenance of improvement.

Co-dependence is an important feature of some patients' current environment. Family or couple interventions can reduce it. Of course, it has been shown that family intervention is invaluable for people with psychosis whose families are over-involved or over-critical (Falloon & Pederson 1985).

Social interventions

Alcoholics Anonymous, Narcotics Anonymous and related groups have been a central plank for community and residential (Twelve Step or Minnesota model) substance misuse recovery for many years. North American dual diagnosis programmes use this approach as part of the therapeutic process. There are many other types of residential rehabilitation provision, including Christian communities, mainly in the non-statutory sector. Similarly, there are many mental health after-care facilities. The two groups of provision do not overlap. Sheltered housing also tends to segregate between mental health and substance misuse.

Biological, psychological and social interventions must be modified to take into account specific dual diagnosis issues. For example, a patient with schizophrenia and alcohol misuse who has significant depressive symptoms probably requires alcohol intervention and possibly modification of antipsy-chotic medication before treating for a depressive illness.

Service planning and resources

Dual diagnosis services, whether 'virtual' or specific teams, require resources at different levels. Such patients are time-consuming and collaborative processes are both essential and costly. Community services (including primary care) must be supported by inpatient facilities with staff oriented to all the clinical issues. Crisis responses should be prepared to deal with these patients and not merely see them as troublesome. Consideration should be given to providing short-term inpatient assessment, detoxification and recovery facilities, if not already present, to allow proper planning of all aspects of treatment and aftercare.

Conclusion

Dual diagnosis treatment requires a high level of diagnostic skill and extensive collaboration. There are significant areas of knowledge, skills and attitudes that must be addressed. There is a significant range of specific interventions that can be used, although they may have to be adapted to this diverse group of patients. All services must adopt a more flexible, 'patient-focused' approach and address reasons why it has been difficult hitherto. The use of a care planning mechanism such as the Care Programme Approach can be helpful and it is essential to use a bio-psychosocial paradigm. Whatever models of service are adopted, there are significant resource implications that cannot be ignored. It is very important to have a range of appropriately oriented facilities, including both community and inpatient components.

References

Bien, T.H., Miller, W.R. & Tonigan, J.S. (1993) Brief interventions for alcohol problems: a review. *Addiction* **88**, 315–336.

Checinski, K. (1998) Depression and alcohol misuse. *Psychiatry Reviews* **3**, 5–10.

Cohen, I.S. (1995) Overdiagnosis of schizophrenia: role of alcohol and drug misuse. *The Lancet* **346**, 1541–1542.

Drake, R.E., Bartels, S.J., Teague, G.B., Noordsy, D.L. & Clark, R.E. (1993) Treatment of substance abuse in severely mentally ill patients. *Journal of Nervous and Mental Disease* **181**, 606–611.

Evans, K. & Sullivan, J.M. (1990) *Dual Diagnosis: Counselling the Mentally Ill Substance Abuser.* Guilford Press, New York.

Falloon, I.R. & Pederson, J. (1985) Family management in the prevention of morbidity of schizophrenia: the adjustment of the family unit. *British Journal of Psychiatry* **147**, 156–163.

Fuller, R.K., Branchey, L., Brightwell, D.R. *et al.* (1986) Disulfiram treatment of alcoholism: A Veterans Administration cooperative study. *Journal of the American Medical Association* **256**, 1449–1455.

Galanter, M., Egelko, S., Edwards, H. & Vergary, M. (1994) A treatment system for combined psychiatric and addictive illness. *Addiction* **89**, 1227–1235.

Ghodse, A.H. (1995) *Drugs and Addictive Behaviour: A Guide to Treatment*, 2nd edn. Blackwell Science, Oxford.

Glautier, S. & Drummond, D.C. (1994) A conditioning approach to the analysis and treatment of drinking problems. *British Medical Bulletin* **50**, 186–199.

Heather, N. & Robertson, I. (1983) *Controlled Drinking*. Cambridge University Press, Cambridge.

Heather, N., Tebbott, J.S., Mattick, R.P. & Zamir, R. (1993) Development of a scale for measuring impaired control over alcohol consumption. *Journal of Studies on Alcohol* **54**, 700–709.

Heather, N., Whitton, B. & Robertson, I. (1986) Evaluation of a self-help manual for media-recruited problem drinkers: six-month follow-up results. *British Journal of Clinical Psychology* **25**, 19–34.

Johnson, S. (1997) Dual diagnosis of severe mental illness and substance misuse: a case for specialist services? *British Journal of Psychiatry* **171**, 205–208.

Kaufman (1994) *Psychotherapy of Addicted Persons*. Guilford Press, New York.

Kemp, R., Hayward, P., Applewhaite, G., Everitt, B. & David, A. (1996) Compliance therapy in psychotic inpatients: randomised controlled trial. *British Medical Journal* **312**, 345–349.

Ley, A., Jeffery, D.P., McLaren, S. & Siegfried, N. (2000) *Treatment Programmes for People with Both Severe Mental Illness and Substance Misuse (Cochrane Review)*S.a a. In: The Cochrane Library, Issue, 1, 2000. Update Software, Oxford.

Lhuitre, J.P., Moore, N. & Tran, G. (1990) Acamprosate appears to decrease alcohol intake in weaned alcoholics. *Alcohol and Alcoholism* **25**, 613–622.

Marlatt, G.A. & Gordon, J.R. (1985) *Relapse Prevention*. Guilford Press, New York.

McInnes, G.T. (1987) Chlormethiazole and alcohol: a lethal cocktail. *BMJ* **294**, 592.

Miller, W.R. (1983) Motivational interviewing with problem drinkers. *Behavioural Psychotherapy* **11**, 147–172.

Miller, W.R. & Rollnick, S. (1991) *Motivational Interviewing: Preparing People to Change Addictive Behaviour*. Guilford Press, New York.

Morland, J., Johnsen, J. & Bache-Wiig, J.E. (1984) Lack of pharmacological effects of implanted disulfiram. In: G. Edwards & J. Littleton (eds) *Pharmacological Treatments for Alcoholism*. Plenum Press, New York.

NHS Management Executive (1994) Health Service Guidelines HSG 94, 27: discharge of mentally disordered people and their continuing care in the community. NHS Executive, London.

O'Malley, S.S., Jaffe, A.J., Chang, G., Schottenfeld, R.S., Meyer, R.E. & Rounsaville, B.J. (1992) Naltrexone and coping skills therapy for alcohol dependence: a controlled trial. *Archives of General Psychiatry* **49**, 881–887.

Rorstad, P. & Checinski, K. (1996) *Dual Diagnosis: Facing the Challenge*. Wynne Howard Publishing, Kenley.

Volpicelli, J.R., Alterman, A.I., Hayashida, M. & O'Brien, C.P. (1992) Naltrexone in the treatment of alcohol dependence. *Archives of General Psychiatry* **49**, 876–880.

Weaver, T., Renton, A., Stimson, G. & Tyrer, P. (1999) Severe mental illness and substance misuse (editorial). *British Medical Journal* **318**, 137–138.

11: Nursing Interventions in the Care of Dually Diagnosed Clients

Peter Price

Introduction

The anecdotal evidence of many mental health nurses and other professionals supports the contention that the problems of working with dually diagnosed clients is a significant issue in contemporary mental health care. In 1997 Gournay *et al.* published a paper highlighting the research evidence for the coexistence of severe mental health problems and substance abuse/dependence, suggesting that such clients were a major challenge for mental health nursing. Since effective working involves both assertive case management for the severely mentally ill as well as specific skills in substance abuse, mental health nurses are in the position of utilising both given the opportunities provided by education and training in psychosocial interventions and case management (Gournay *et al.* 1997).

The recognition of the problems presented to professionals in working with clients with a dual diagnosis is often complicated by ideologies related to both models of treatment and the most effective methods of treatment. These issues relate to the way in which care and treatment are organised and delivered, and as such cloud judgements about the most effective approaches that promote the most successful outcomes. It is stated that generic mental health care teams often lack experience, knowledge, skills and confidence in dealing with the dually diagnosed, while staff in addiction services may consider the existence of psychoses to be beyond their remit and their generally challenging approach not suited to such clients (Johnson 1997; Gafoor & Rassool 1998). Furthermore attempts to integrate the care provided by two distinct services may only fragment an approach to clients who are difficult to engage and require consistency and continuity of care. With the help of further evaluative studies (Ley *et al.* 1999), this is an issue for service planners.

Evidence has emerged from the USA in recent years of the effectiveness of providing continuity of care by the integration of treatment for clients with severe mental illnesses and substance misuse problems (Drake *et al.* 1996; Mueser *et al.* 1998). Integrated treatment programmes share essential elements—assertive outreach, comprehensiveness, shared decision making, long-term commitment, stage-wise treatment, pharmacotherapy—and these elements thread their way throughout the total programme of care and treatment. Integrated treatment is often based upon abstinence rather than controlled use, and the concept of treatment in stages derives from recognition that changes in maladaptive behaviour patterns occur in different stages (Mahoney 1991). Recognising these stages give clinicians clues as to which interventions are more likely to be successful at a particular point in the treatment process.

This chapter aims to offer some structure to the overall process of care, discuss the type of cognitive interventions that may be used during the stages of care, and recognise some of the potential pitfalls inherent in caring for this client group. A case study will illustrate the complex problems associated with dual diagnosis.

A framework for therapeutic interventions

Osher and Kofoed (1989) describe four stages of *engagement, persuasion, active treatment*, and *relapse prevention*, and these provide a useful framework for utilising therapeutic interventions. Within these stages exist various cognitive approaches to the care and treatment of clients, such as family education and problem solving, persuasion, motivational interviewing, individual cognitive behavioural counselling, lifestyle changes and relapse planning and prevention. Active treatment, the third of Osher and Kofoed's four stages is multifaceted, and will vary from patient to patient, but the other three will now be considered in general terms, followed by an examination of some of the underlying cognitive approaches.

Engagement

The lack of a working alliance between the client and nurse is the hallmark of the engagement stage of care and treatment. Attempts to establish a therapeutic relationship prematurely exacerbate the potential for dropping out before real treatment has commenced. Nurses typically undertake outreach work that includes practical help with food and shelter, social support and intervening in crises. The aim is to understand the client and their view, to respond to their behaviour and language, to recognise their often unspoken needs, and thereby to develop some trust and genuineness. This demands skill, patience and perseverance, and nurses who are not equipped both personally and interpersonally to undertake it should steer well clear. Substance misuse is not addressed directly until the end of the engagement process when a working alliance has developed.

Persuasion

The persuasion stage offers the first real opportunity to use structured cognitive approaches in the care of dually diagnosed clients, and is contingent upon regular contact and a working alliance between clinician and client. In this context persuasion is about empowering the client to gain the insight and to have the desire and strength for change. At this stage many clients still do not view their substance misuse as problematic or attempt to modify their behaviour. Essentially they are still unmotivated. Strategies include motivational interviewing, individual and family education, the use of persuasion, sampling and review of alternative social and recreational activities, and initial preparation for lifestyle changes to achieve successful abstinence.

Relapse and relapse prevention

It is not uncommon for clients to return to substance use during active treatment and it is best to see this as part of the process of a chronic illness. Both client and nurse must accept relapse and move on rather than experiencing it as failure and giving in to it. Many clients will have opted for a reduced or controlled use of substances during the early treatment stage. Often this is doomed to failure, but in the long term their experience of it will enable them to see that abstinence is the more viable and profitable option. Working together both client and nurse can review the possible causes, antecedents and triggers, considering new areas for change and enhancing old ones. If the substance use is more than a slip—in other words it is sustained use—a return to the persuasion stage is necessary, whereby the client is once again encouraged and empowered to display their motivation for change.

A period of abstinence from use of substances often results in the client having the confidence to believe that they can resume controlled use. This stage is reached after six months wherein the negative effects of substance use have not been experienced. Once again this is invariably unsuccessful since it is unlikely that clients with severe mental illness will *not* experience such negative effects. Consequently goals of care include maintaining the awareness that relapse is still a real possibility that should be prepared for, and to expand recovery activities into other areas of life such as relationships, work, and health. Nurses should enable and encourage clients to continue to attend specific and self-help groups, utilise other community support networks, attend individual sessions to review their progress and difficulties and receive support, and to maintain commitment to newly established family relationships and ways of communicating.

This illustrates how a shift in focus from abstinence from substance use into other areas of life functioning is necessary. Giving up substances cannot be the ultimate and enduring focus for the therapeutic relationship, and the client should be helped to move towards other goals such as normative relationships, employment and leisure activities. The nurse has a role in identifying and arranging supported employment as well as undertaking or arranging social skills training to enhance the opportunity for success. Specific issues for social skills training include starting and maintaining conversations, refusing offers of alcohol and drugs from others, challenging self defeating cognitions, how to express negative feelings appropriately and actively seeking out other leisure activities. As well as giving homework to clients, it is of vital importance that there are planned methods to generalise acquired behaviours into the client's real environment. A case study is presented later in the chapter to highlight the complex problems in dealing with dual diagnosis clients and the application of appropriate therapeutic interventions.

Motivational interviewing

Miller and Rollnick (1994) characterised motivation as something that one *does* rather than has. It is essential first to recognise a problem and then look for a way to change. Once a strategy for change is identified the problem is then to begin the change and to stick with it.

Empathy is the ability to communicate to the client an understanding of their experience and their world and is evident in verbal and non-verbal behaviour. Active listening skills such as eye contact, body posture and facial expression convey understanding of the client's situation, and particular skill may be needed here bearing in mind the potential misinterpretation of intent by the client related to their prevailing mental status. Skilful reflecting back of the client's thoughts, fears, doubts and hopes add to an atmosphere of genuineness, trust and empathy. It is important at this stage not to offer advice, give judgement, or attempt to question or teach ways of dealing with needs and problems. These skills are clearly within the repertoire of mental health and specialist addiction nurses.

Careful questioning may reveal a *discrepancy* between the situation that the client is currently in and where they wish to be. Developing this discrepancy by exploring personal goals and considering what steps are necessary to achieve these encourage motivation for change. Clients may be asked to describe the possible consequences of their substance use, and nurses may selectively use reflective listening to reinforce the recognition that substance use adversely affects attainment of personal goals.

Arguing with the client at this stage serves only to strengthen their beliefs and attitudes towards their substance use, the opposite of what the nurse is hoping to achieve. The reasons for behaviour change should be acknowledged and stated by the client and not the clinician. Resistance to change is rooted in ambivalence, and it is important to view such ambivalence as normal and not pathological. Resistance should be explored rather than opposed, the key being to *roll with resistance* rather than combat it.

Optimism and hope are essential to any change process and the nurse should show his/her confidence in change being possible. The client will have experienced successes and frustrations in the past, and exploring positive aspects may produce a positive focus for the future. Acknowledging and *supporting the client's self-efficacy* may increase motivation for change.

Motivational interviewing may produce positive results over time if conducted skilfully. Traps such as using confrontation will produce denial; being the expert and labelling the client will prove counterproductive; indulging in question and answer type formats may defeat the object of enabling the client to recognise the negative effects of their substance misuse themselves. The nurse should always employ open-ended questions, reflective listening, and summarising of what the client has said. Affirming positive contributions and the enhancing self-motivational statements are essential elements of this process.

Individual cognitive behavioural counselling

Cognitive behavioural therapy has been shown to be a potent therapeutic tool for a range of mental health problems (Dattilio & Freeman 1992). This is no less true in dually diagnosed clients, where the skilful use of analysis, disputing cognitions, combined with realistic homework tasks can enhance the skills that promote abstinence including increasing self-efficacy in finding, establishing and maintaining appropriate support networks. Such work should not occur until clients are actively engaged in the care and treatment process.

A functional analysis may be undertaken with the client, examining positive and negative consequences of using or not using substances. For example, positive consequences for using may include the alleviation of symptoms and boredom, socialisation, pleasure and recreation; negative consequences may include conflict, legal, financial and housing problems, risk of contracting sexually transmitted and other diseases (HIV, Hepatitis B and C), as well as symptom exacerbation and relapse. Conversely, the positive consequences of not using substances may be less conflict and better relationships, stable housing, and reduced or absent legal and financial problems. If the client were to cease to use substances the negative consequences may be viewed as less opportunity for socialisation and recreation, intractable boredom, and perceived difficulty in coping with symptoms and other problems of living. Invariably these areas are based upon the individual's unique past history and the problems they have experienced.

The way the client thinks about their situation influences their potentially negative view of the difficulties presented by abstinence, and the skilled nurse may offer them an alternative frame of reference that may promote success. For example, use of the '100 people technique' (Lam & Gale 2000) can enable the client to move from a subjective and concrete view of their situation towards one that acknowledges their individuality and the possibilities of success.

Family education and problem solving

Families are often integral to the processes of both the mental disorder and substance misuse of the client, and it is therefore wise to involve them in the stages of treatment, and invite them to act as members of the treatment team (Mueser & Glynn 1995). Families who are in contact with the client experience a higher care-giving burden, and loss of family support often destabilises the housing situation of the client, which in turn may lead to greater vulnerability. Family conflict, often unresolved, as well as criticism and hostility provide a trigger for the continued use of psychoactive substances and maintenance of symptoms, and working upon communication patterns and coping skills can act to reduce this. The structured use of time in order to decrease the opportunities for drug misuse, and simple behavioural rewards for achieving set goals are important positive effects that can be met within families who may spend more time with the client than the nurse. Invariably both the client and family members benefit from education about the mental disorder, substances and substance abuse, interactions between the two, and the principles of the treatment programme embarked upon. At this stage it is important to have established that it is the client him- or herself that wants to make the change, and not simply as a result of family or nurse pressure.

As well as empathy and support, nurses may provide forms of practical support such as with benefits, transport, resolving immediate problems, and childminding arrangements. As with the client the family needs to be gradually engaged, and in the long term an aim may be to enable all family members to reduce their stress, improve their lives, and develop their own support networks. Families are in a prime position to encourage compliance with prescribed drugs and to monitor usage of illicit ones, especially if relapse has occurred, as well as to set limits upon behaviour. Involvement is long-term, and eventually the move may be made from single to group family work. Apart from the obvious economic advantages the family will benefit from broader peer, social and therapeutic support and be less vulnerable to the negative effects of ongoing staff changes. In family group meetings the nurse acts initially as a leader and educator, moving to the role of facilitator as the involvement of the families increases. Nurses should clearly focus upon present and future goals, and not on the past.

Case study 1

Tom is in his mid thirties, and has a history of schizophrenia and poly-drug misuse that includes cannabis, ecstasy, amphetamines and occasionally cocaine as well as alcohol. He has a history of criminality including burglary and violence and has been in prison for a total of 18 months. For the past 15 years he has had numerous hospital admissions for relapse of his illness, each time returning to the care of the community psychiatric services.

Tom lives alone in his own flat but is rarely found there, preferring to spend his time on the streets with his friends or with a casual partner with whom he has an 8-year-old daughter. He rarely sees his parents, although they express concern about him. He is difficult to track down, and when he can be found he declines any engagement in the care and treatment process saying that this is the life he wants to live.

Continued on p. 154.

A community psychiatric nurse (CPN) was assigned to Tom's case, the initial task being to engage him in the care and treatment process. He was befriended at his known haunts – the local park, near an off-licence, occasionally at his flat. The emphasis was upon getting to know him and offering practical help such as arranging visits to see his daughter, telephone contact with his parents, helping him to meet his dietary needs, arranging for him to see his GP when he contracted conjunctivitis, and offering a contact number to call in times of crisis.

The CPN attempted to talk in ways that he could relate to, and not to be judgemental, prescriptive or unreliable, until gradually they were seen to be an increasing part of Tom's social world. At this point he would sometimes seek out the nurse to ask for advice or help on a variety of matters, such as access to his daughter and the possible effects of a drug he had been offered. This point was considered to be an appropriate time to move tentatively towards the next stage of persuading Tom of the potential benefits of behaviour change away from substance abuse and towards abstinence.

Tom felt that at present he was stuck in an existence that offered little prospect except more of the same. Although he liked his friends and his lifestyle he saw that they were preventing him from stabilising his relationship with his daughter, partner and parents, as well as the possibility of leading him back into hospital and into prison, which he definitely did not want. He tended to deny that his substance misuse impacted upon his mental illness and could exacerbate the symptoms, but acknowledged that it could be significant in the financial problems that plagued him. When asked to describe the ultimate consequences of his substance misuse, Tom was able to reflect and offer 'death' as the only option, adding that he did not care. He initially refuted any notion that he could possibly alter such a chain of events, as he had seen two of his friends die from substance misuse. Rather than contest the incorrect assumption that it was inevitable, the nurse demonstrated empathy with the acknowledgement that it must be very difficult for Tom, whilst offering the optimistic view that he could determine his own future if he really wanted to with some help. For the first time Tom said that he had succeeded in stopping taking drugs for a year in the past without any help. The nurse was able to explore this success with him in terms of his actions and the benefits he felt, and this opportunity provided a catalyst with which to secure some commitment on his part for behaviour change.

Tom's view of his need for substances hinged on the idea that he could not live without them because they provided pleasure, companionship and escape from psychiatric symptoms. Talk of giving up made him feel uncomfortable and anxious because he could not see how he could possibly survive without them. The nurse was able to explore ways of living without drugs, and to suggest how he might reasonably assert his feelings and thoughts positively when negotiating prescribed drug treatments

Continued.

with his doctor. They were able to discuss ideas of equality and democracy in friendship, and how he had many likeable characteristics such as a good sense of humour and concern for others (notably his daughter). It was suggested that Tom could form relationships with others that did not revolve around substance misuse, and he agreed that he might try some social skills training to achieve this end.

Tom's unhelpful thinking about the ways in which substance misuse affected him made him susceptible to others' demands, and expectations that he could not control fuelled his continued use. The nurse aimed to alter his perception of himself to show that he had choices about how he viewed situations and the negative feelings they engendered in him. For example, if he was offered drugs he felt compelled to accept because if he declined he would be rejected by the group which he would find difficult to deal with because these were the only people who would accept him. In other words he felt that he only had value within this group and he was worthless outside, unable to see any way to refuse and maintain face. The nurse explored this with him, asking how he thought others might refuse to buy drugs, could there be another way he could view his situation, for example he might be a stronger person than others by refusing. Tom needed much work on his self-esteem and assertiveness, and gradually the skilful use of cognitive counselling approaches empowered him to see that substance misuse and the possible consequences of it were not inevitable for him.

Tom's contact with his parents, partner and daughter was not regular, although he would have liked it to be more so. The nurse made appointments with both his parents and partner to obtain their views and enlist their support and participation in his care and treatment. It was clear that they did care about Tom, and encouraged by his attempts at change agreed to participate as best they could. It is of course not always as straightforward, especially when partners are also involved in substance misuse.

Both required some understanding of his psychiatric illness, his particular substance misuse, how the two interacted, and how these were directly related to the problems he found himself in. Furthermore, a full explanation of the treatment process and their place in it was given. For example, they could encourage his successes, monitor his use of illicit and prescribed drugs, offer him sanctuary and alternative activities particularly at times of vulnerability, and not subject him to negative and hostile comments which might result in continual relapse. Here nurses must employ the full range of psycho-educational interventions to maximise the therapeutic potential of enlisting the family in the care process.

In conjunction with Tom the nurse arranged regular (at least once weekly) visits to see his partner and daughter. It was agreed that these co-

Continued on p. 156.

Continued.

incided with shopping time, so that the three of them could spend the time together in normal activities. Similarly Tom's parents agreed to invite him for lunch, possibly with his partner and daughter, once a month. They agreed to report Tom's illicit and prescribed drug usage, as well as significant changes in his behaviour. In time his partner said she would consider attending group family meetings. Tom regularly attended the active treatment groups as well as individual counselling sessions. At the same time he was keen to keep up regular appointments with his doctor, who carefully titrated his dosage of antipsychotic medication to keep symptoms and side-effects to a minimum. With all going well for some months the danger of relapse increased as he now felt that he had control of the problem and could use substances socially and selectively. Fortunately in his case relapse did not constitute sustained use, but the nurse had to return to the persuasion stage to empower Tom to see that in his case controlled use was not an option. Discussion also explored the ways in which Tom might expand his activities in other ways, such as exercise, hobbies and interests, and paid employment.

Although long-term engagement and therapeutic work is essential Tom remains in contact with the psychiatric services and his quality of life has improved considerably. He sees his parents, partner and daughter regularly, and continues to contribute to the active treatment group. It has not been easy and in total he has had three relapses. Importantly his treatment team has remained relatively stable and has maintained a positive and optimistic therapeutic stance.

Conclusion

Despite the fact that education and training for working with this client group is limited in the United Kingdom, it is important to recognise that many mental health and specialist addiction nurses already possess some of the skills essential for effective working. As the most numerous of any professional grouping in mental health care it is important that nurses accept the challenge of working with the dually diagnosed. Many will already possess some of the person-centred skills necessary for effective care, and where limitations are evident they may seek further education and training to remedy this. Individual nurses may use these on an individual basis, but it is desirable that they are recognised and harnessed in the planning of care at service level. Until this happens nurses who are in the forefront of care have a duty to employ contemporary and effective skills in their care and treatment. A structured process that includes cognitive interventions offers just such opportunity for this.

Notwithstanding the problems and challenges presented by dually diagnosed clients there can be some hope for their care and treatment. Although such people can often be difficult and frustrating to work with it is an enviable strength of mental health nurses that they can always find positive and endearing characteristics in their clients, and this should not be lost on service planners. Interventions that are matched to the state of client motivation at any one time, and that are person-centred and flexible in response to need offer hope for successfully treating what is often a miserable existence for the sufferer. The skill of mental health nurses in delivering cognitive interventions to such clients is a vital aspect of the care spectrum for a contemporary and challenging health care issue.

References

Dattilio, F.M. & Freeman, A. (1992) Introduction to cognitive therapy. In: A. Freeman & F.M. Dattilio (eds) *Comprehensive Casebook of Cognitive Therapy*. Plenum Press, New York.

Drake, R.E., Mueser, K.T., Clark, R.E. *et al.* (1996) The course, treatment and outcome of substance disorder in persons with severe mental illness. *American Journal of Orthopsychiatry* **66**, 42–51.

Gafoor, M. & Rassool, G. Hussein (1998) The co-existence of psychiatric disorders and substance misuse: working with dual diagnosis patients. *Journal of Advanced Nursing* **27**, 497–502.

Gournay, K., Sandford, T., Johnson, S. & Thornicroft, G. (1997) Dual diagnosis of severe mental health problems and substance abuse/dependence: a major priority for mental health nursing. *Journal of Psychiatric and Mental Health Nursing* **4**, 89–95.

Johnson, S. (1997) Dual diagnosis of severe mental illness and substance misuse: a case for specialist services. *British Journal of Psychiatry* **171**, 205–208.

Lam, D. & Gale, J. (2000) Cognitive Behaviour Therapy: teaching a client the ABC model—the first step towards the process of change. *Journal of Advanced Nursing* **31** (2), 444–451.

Ley, A., Jeffery, D.P., McLaren, S. & Siegfried, N. (1999) Treatment programmes for people with both severe mental illness and substance misuse. The Cochrane Library (Oxford), Issue 3.

Mahoney, M.J. (1991) Human change processes. *The Scientific Foundations of Psychotherapy*. Basic Books, Delran, NJ.

Miller, W.R. & Rollnick, S. (1994) *Motivational Interviewing. Preparing People to Change Addictive Behaviour*. Guilford Press, New York.

Mueser, K.T., Drake, R.E. & Noordsy, D.L. (1998) Integrated mental health and substance abuse treatment for severe psychiatric disorders. *Journal of Practical Psychology and Behavioral Health* **4** (3), 129–139.

Mueser, K.T. & Glynn, S.M. (1995) Families as members of the treatment team. In: *Behavioural Family Therapy for Psychiatric Disorders* (Ch. 1). Allyn & Bacon, Needham Heights, MA.

Osher, F.C. & Kofoed, L.L. (1989) Treatment of patients with psychiatric and psychoactive substance abuse disorders. *Hospital Community Psychiatry* **40**, 1025–1030.

12: Brief Strategic Therapy — Working with the Patient's Motivation for Change

Vivienne Saunders

Introduction

The cycle of change model (Prochaska and Di Clemente 1986) incorporating motivational interviewing (Miller & Rollnick 1991) and relapse prevention (Marlatt & Gordon 1985) have been proved to benefit many patients at certain stages of their drug using career. The 12-step Alcoholics Anonymous model undoubtedly provides a self-help solution for others. Some patients do not respond to either model yet it is common for health care professionals to keep trying, offering more of the same treatment that has not helped, we have even given the phenomenon a name — 'the revolving door' — to describe the same patients entering the same treatment facility again and again. It is common to alleviate our frustration by blaming the patient for the failure of the treatment, we say he/she is 'in denial', 'dysfunctional', or 'has not yet touched bottom'. When people are unable to change their behaviour they resort to explaining it, the same is true of professionals.

Brief Strategic Therapy (BST) focuses on solutions and uses the strengths and resources of the patient rather than concentrating on weaknesses and deficits. Solution focused therapy emerged from the family therapy tradition in the USA, in particular the work of Steve de Shazer in the 1980s. It is certainly not intended to present this type of therapy as a total solution but as an alternative or a useful tool to be incorporated into traditional treatments.

Brief Strategic Therapy

The working definition of Brief Strategic Therapy is a therapy, which makes the maximum impact within a rationed amount of time. The prominent features of any brief therapy which focuses on solutions have been characterised by Barret-Kruse (1994) as:

- The view that self and colleagues are essentially able.
- The acceptance of the patient's definition of the problem.
- The formation of the therapeutic alliance.
- The crediting of success to the patient.
- The therapist learning from the patient.
- The avoidance of a power struggle with the patient.

- The objectification, rather than the personalisation of the patient's behaviour.

Positive change is expected by the therapist and communicated to the patient, the formation of the therapeutic alliance is assumed from the outset and the therapist is directive (e.g. in setting homework tasks). It is sometimes assumed that all therapy with mentally ill patients will be long term and that substance misuse is a relapsing condition also indicating long-term treatment. This need not mean that effective treatment of patients with a dual diagnosis takes twice as long.

BST essentially focuses on the present and the future, clear attainable goals are set and the therapist is openly influential and experienced by the patient as confident, hopeful and competent. This therapy is designed to be intermittent throughout the patient's life and can be resumed at points of crisis. There is evidence to suggest that brief therapy is the choice of the consumer, many patients want to 'go through' treatment rather than be 'in treatment'. There have been many studies which demonstrate that brief therapy is as effective as long-term therapy and that the former is the preference of 70% of patients (Garfield & Bergin 1994). Hoyt (1994) makes the point that 'More is not necessarily better. Better is better'. That success can be accomplished rapidly is true, but this does not mean that it is an easy process.

It is important to talk about what the patient wants to have present in their lives (the solution) rather than just the absence of the problem. By sticking closely to the patient's agenda the therapist enables the patient to focus on the attainable rather than being daunted by the enormity of the problem. The author's clinical work is based in general practice, the patients being referred to me by members of the primary health care team. It should be noted that my remit covers all psychotropic substances and that if the patient referred has any diagnosed mental illness they are defined by the GP as 'stable'. The case example which follows is an illustration of BST being used with a dual diagnosis patient in the general practice setting.

Case study 2

Anne, aged 53, was referred by her GP for smoking cessation therapy and anxiety management. Common aetiological factors were believed to be responsible for the onset of her mental illness (anxiety and depression) and substance misuse (tobacco, cannabis and alcohol). She had complex physical as well as psychiatric problems and the GP practice nurse and CPN variously described her as 'a heart sink patient', 'charming', 'exasperating', 'good fun' and 'hopeless'.

Continued on p. 160.

Continued.

Background

When she was 40 Anne had a riding accident which injured her spine. She spent some months in a wheelchair before graduating to walking with the aid of sticks. Around this time she experienced her first depression which became severe and she was admitted for inpatient treatment. She was discharged after two months and appeared to do well until about five years ago when she presented to her general practitioner with a variety of symptoms. He referred her to the community mental health team and she was diagnosed as suffering from panic disorder and depression. Anne was prescribed diazepam and amitriptyline, which had worked well previously. Withdrawal from the benzodiazepines after 12 months continuous use had proved difficult and rebound anxiety was experienced. Two referrals had been made to anxiety management groups and Anne had completed both courses with little lasting success. She had attended a hospital based smoking cessation service six months ago and had quit for two weeks before relapsing. The practice nurse had been treating her for smoking cessation and the community psychiatric nurse (CPN) for relaxation therapy since, but without noticeable improvement. Recently the CPN had smelt alcohol on Anne's breath and warned the patient that she was drinking at a hazardous level. Referral to a specialist alcohol team had been offered.

Anne was defined by her GP as a somatiser. Some of her disorders had a true physical pathology partly induced by stress (essential hypertension, and eczema) and some which did not resulted from anatomical disturbance (tension headaches, hyperventilation and irritable bowel syndrome). It is the latter that DSM-V classifies as 'somatisation disorder' in which anxiety and depression have a direct effect. The professionals (GP, practice nurse, CPN and surgeon) involved in her care all agreed that smoking was exacerbating her physical problems. Anne herself was very keen to give up prior to having an operation on her spine which, it was hoped, would improve her mobility and alleviate pain.

Therapeutic interventions

BST does not spend time building a rapport with the patient, it assumes it. Anne accepted readily that she had not come to talk about the past and that it was necessary for her to define her present problem(s). She said that she was 'desperate' to quit smoking but had been unable to do so because it was the only thing that alleviated her anxiety. Asked what her therapeutic goal was Anne explained that there had to be two, to quit smoking and not to be anxious. The long-term BST goal was her vision of a life not disabled by anxiety (as apart from the utopian goal of being free of any anxious thoughts). The interim goal, i.e. the goal of the therapy, was to quit smoking and learn effective methods of managing anxiety. Each session would have a specific goal moving towards the interim goal. Anne found this strange in that she had not considered that once started towards her goal she would be able to manage the rest of the way herself. It is more usual to examine past mistakes, things that did not work, in the hope that patient and therapist will learn from them. To maintain optimism it was explained that we would focus only on things that did work or had helped.

It is necessary to discover how maladaptive coping strategies have maintained the problem. Anne described an almost continuous state of anxiety indicative of the somewhat controversial diagnosis of 'generalised anxiety disorder' with her constant worrying, mostly about her health. As well as this 'free floating' anxiety there was evidence of panic disorder as defined by DSM-IV. She described this as suddenly becoming intensely frightened, she would gasp for breath and feel that her heart was about to burst out of her chest, she experienced abdominal pain became very cold and was certain that she was having a heart attack. Her coping strategy was to light a cigarette and as she inhaled the panic would subside. She said that she felt that she was going mad, as she did not seriously believe that smoking a cigarette could prevent cardiac arrest!

She had been told that when she panicked she hyperventilated and was taught the technique of breathing into a paper bag to prevent this. She understood why this should help, but could not do it by herself. As she told herself to relax she would become increasingly anxious. Some months ago Anne had discovered that alcohol helped her to relax. This was no longer the case, alcohol only 'worked' when taken in conjunction with cannabis, but she had continued to drink in the hope that the initial relief would be repeated.

Definition of the problem—B.S.A.I.C.I.D. profile

Behaviour

The unwanted behavioural response was an attempt to control anxiety by smoking. The symptoms developed five years ago and became exacerbated as each attempt at anxiety management or smoking cessation failed. The symptoms tended not to occur, or not as badly when the patient was with other people. The key to the problem lay in the attempted solution, i.e. smoking increased Anne's anxiety about her health. Telling herself to relax increased the level of anxiety.

Affective response

Anne's emotional response was guilt, she said she 'ought' to be able to manage her anxiety. Her feelings were of increased anxiety and panic. The attempted behavioural solution of self-medication: tobacco, alcohol and cannabis was maladaptive.

161

Sensations

The physical sensations experienced were always negative and accompanied by clinical symptoms (sweating, palpitation, etc.).

Imagery

Anne's image of herself in the past was of a frail, helpless woman. In the present she saw herself as a mixture of weakness and determination. Her image of herself in the future was sometimes as a confident non-smoker and sometimes of 'a nervous wreck'.

Cognition

Anne's self talk when anxious ran along the lines of telling herself to relax. She believed that this should work and that it would work 'for any sane person'. Her idea that she could have a life totally free from anxiety was irrational.

Interpersonal

The patient had no family but had recently joined the local church community and this had enabled her to develop a social life. She had made some close friends whom she experienced as supportive. Anne was unable to practice the relaxation techniques she had been taught because she experienced the locus of control as being with the therapist who had taught them, i.e. they could only work in the therapist's presence.

Drugs

It is essential to screen accurately for total substance misuse at the first consultation. In Anne's case this amounted to:
- 25–30 cigarettes per day
- 4 bottles of table wine (75 cL each) per week (total 36 units of alcohol)
- prescribed medication: fluoxetine (Prozac) 20 mg daily; coproxamol for pain, taken occasionally, never more than 6 tablets per day
- 3.5 g of marijuana per week.

During this session several important facts emerged and became clear to Anne. Anxiety was not the real problem, the real problem was the way she attempted to relieve it, i.e. smoking, which made her feel worse about herself, and telling herself to relax which in fact turned up the anxiety. Cannabis and to a more limited extent alcohol, masked the unpleasant psychological feelings. (Anne had never attempted to disguise her cannabis use, she had simply never been asked about it.)

The patient's problems were rephrased in a positive way; the diagnosis of 'panic attacks' emphasised the problem, so a positive physical explanation of the 'flight or fight response' was given. Anne welcomed this biological explanation as it lessened her fears that she was going mad. The unpleasant symptoms were given a positive connotation, i.e. her body was protecting her from possible danger, she did after all live on a notorious housing estate where muggings and break-ins were common. The utopian goal of never experiencing anxiety was reframed to allow for 'appropriate' or 'manageable' levels. Her belief that she could not stop smoking until she felt better was challenged. BST works on making small incremental changes based on exceptions to the problem and answers to the miracle question:

The miracle question

THERAPIST: 'Let me ask you a strange question that many people find helpful.

ANNE: 'Okay.

THERAPIST: 'Imagine that when you go to sleep tonight a miracle happens and the problems we have been talking about disappear. As you were asleep you did not know that a miracle had happened, when you wake up what would be the first sign that the problems no longer existed?

ANNE: 'Well, I wouldn't even think about smoking, I just wouldn't want a cigarette or a drink, or anything. Yes, I'd have no drugs at all in me and I'd feel really well and, you know, confident.

THERAPIST: 'That sounds good. Tell me, who would be the first person to notice a miracle has happened?

ANNE: 'That would be my best friend, Lynn.

THERAPIST: 'How would you know that she had found out?

ANNE: 'She'd be smiling at me instead of asking me how I am with that dreadful concerned look on her face. She wouldn't be feeling sorry for me; she'd really want to be with me.'

The answer to the miracle question surprised Anne, she said she had not realised until she said it that she really wanted to be drug free. The significance of this was that she stopped insisting that she could not stop smoking until she no longer felt anxious. She was also able to acknowledge that her preoccupation with her health was distancing her from the very people that she wanted to be close to.

This patient found it difficult to accept that nothing lasts forever and that there must be times when the problem was not present.

THERAPIST: 'Perhaps there are times when you have got a little way towards the miracle?

ANNE: 'Well no, I feel bad all the time.

THERAPIST: 'What precisely do you mean by "bad"?

ANNE: 'Guilty, I smoke all the time, I always have drugs rattling or sloshing around inside me.

THERAPIST: 'Always?

ANNE (laughing): 'Not really. I know I won't have any cannabis for a couple of weeks, the bloke I buy from is going on holiday. Oh yes, and I haven't had a drink since that nurse said I should be treated for alcoholism!'

Change prior to the first session

Anne had missed how significant this control over her behaviour was. Like many patients she had made a huge step towards changing her behaviour in between making the first appointment and keeping it. She had so much resented the CPN's view of her alcohol consumption that she had stopped drinking. The professional's potential solution matched the problem, i.e. attending a specialist alcohol service in order for Anne to concentrate on dealing with her drinking. Anne's own solution did not match the problem, she deliberately became more involved in church activities so that she spent little time alone at home. This seemingly unrelated solution broke the drinking pattern and prevented potential addiction. It was not Anne's intention to remain abstinent, her goal was to not drink at all for two weeks and then not to drink when she was alone. This amounted to sharing a bottle of wine with her friend, once a week.

Frequent experience of relapse makes it difficult for professionals working in the field of addiction to accept that people can and do take charge of their drinking. Negative experience no doubt encourages a degree of scepticism yet there is no research to support the belief that dual diagnosis patients cannot control their drinking. What was important in Anne's case was that she believed she had control, and she was likely to be successful because she had worked out for herself where she wanted to be on a scale of controlled drinking. Anne had no symptoms of physical dependency; blood tests revealed her gamma GT and MCV levels remained normal.

Potential problems

It was important to check out what specifically Anne meant by being drug free as those involved in her care felt it essential that she continued to take her antidepressants. Anne saw a future free of depression but understood being taken off her prescribed medication was a very long-term goal. She was hopeful that the proposed operation would mean that she took fewer painkillers, but this was in the medium-term future. Anne was confident that any problem with alcohol was already in the past but the information she had just received that smoking any substance is injurious to health was most unwelcome. Getting into an argument about her cannabis use would have been counterproductive and she was left to consider this aspect further, particularly that continuing to smoke cannabis was likely to impact negatively on the smoking cessation intervention.

Smoking cessation treatment

There was little doubt that this patient was nicotine dependent as she fulfilled the main criteria, i.e. smoked more than 10 cigarettes a day, lit up within half an hour of waking and smoked if she woke up during the night. In addition she found the habit of smoking very comforting, she experienced her last attempt to give up as similar to suffering bereavement. She made the decision to use nicotine replacement therapy as research shows that this would double her chance of success. This would avoid the physical symptoms of withdrawal whilst she coped with the loss of the smoking habit and learnt other ways of controlling her anxiety. Methods of nicotine replacement were discussed and she chose to use the transdermal 24 h patch. It was expected and accepted that she would benefit from a three-month reduction course with motivational support being provided in general practice. At her first consultation Anne registered a count of 42 on the carbon monoxide monitor.

Anxiety management

Anne had unrealistic expectations in regard to managing her anxiety; she was seeking something magical that would take it away. Many attempts had been made to find the root cause of the panic attacks yet it is not necessary to fully understand the past to positively influence the present and the future. Just as the unpleasant symptoms did not arrive fully formed (a recognisable firing pattern had emerged), so remission would not arrive fully formed either. Anne could see that the anxiety attacks did in fact have a beginning, middle and, most importantly an end. Her past therapy had taken the premise that people do not learn when they are anxious and emphasised that the patient must be relaxed in order to learn new ways of coping. But Anne had learnt to panic when she was anxious and SFT needs the patient to be highly stimulated if re-education is to take place. Scaling is a technique, which brings this re-education about.

Scaling

THERAPIST: 'On a scale of nought to 10, nought representing no anxiety and 10 the most anxious you have ever been, where would you place yourself now?

ANNE: 'About 5.

THERAPIST: 'That's good. Now I would like you to sit back, resting both feet on the floor, your hands comfortably on your thighs. When you are ready perhaps you will gently allow your eyes to close . . . Keep breathing in the way that we have practised . . . that's right, breathe through your nose, keeping your mouth closed . . . good . . . Pay full attention to your body, at first the outside, your skin . . . then gradually becoming more aware of the inside of you . . . noticing the temperature . . . any sensations, any feelings . . . as you continue to scan your body, just becoming aware of any areas of tension . . . or worry . . . becoming aware of how sensitive you are to your body . . . Be aware of where in your body you are experiencing that tension . . . I would like you to continue to experience those feelings . . . Where on the scale are you now?

ANNE: 'About 7, no 8.

THERAPIST: 'Isn't that interesting how you can continue to explore those feelings, having the courage to experience them . . . You know often things can get a little worse before they get better . . . you are observing the process . . . (Long pause) where on the scale are you now?

ANNE: (very long pause) 'It's falling, falling back to 5.

THERAPIST: 'Interesting how that feeling takes care of itself when you allow yourself to experience it . . . allowing it to pass . . . Just allow the process to continue for a while . . . (long pause) Where are you now?

ANNE: 'Fine, about a 2.

THERAPIST: 'Fine, perhaps you will slide deeper . . . maybe to nought . . . or even into minus . . .

ANNE: 'I'm still at 2.

THERAPIST: 'Maybe that's a comfortable place to be right now.

ANNE: 'Yes.

THERAPIST: 'When you are ready bring your attention back . . . becoming aware of sitting comfortably in the chair . . . the heaviness fading away . . . Gently, very gently, allow your eyes to open . . . aware of feeling alert and refreshed . . .'

Anne was surprised that she had relaxed without the word being mentioned. Since a perception that it is the therapist not the patient who is in control will almost certainly lead to relapse, it was necessary to point out that she had only been encouraged to stay with whatever feeling she was experiencing. She said that she had started to go through a typical initial period of self-doubt and worry and the physical sensations of anxiety had mounted. She was pleased that this had come to a natural end without recourse to smoking.

Homework

The setting of homework tasks is an integral part of BST. Anne was reminded that the periods between sessions had to be used and she was willing to do this. Her quit day for smoking was set for the next day. She was asked to practise worrying for 15 minutes a day. During this time she would avoid hyperventilation by breathing through her nose with her mouth closed. If anxiety occurred during these worry periods she would welcome it as an opportunity to practice the scaling technique she had learnt in the session. At the end of the worry period she would make brief notes and bring them to her next session. Her main concern was that 15 minutes was too short a time for a whole day's worrying but she agreed to stick to the plan.

Before the next session Anne consulted her GP about a physical problem and told him that she did not think the therapy was working. I had told her to worry for 15 minutes a day and it had not worked. She had followed the instruction for the first four days with success. On the fifth day she could only manage 5 minutes and she had not been able to worry at all that day!

Outcome

Anne quit smoking as planned. Her carbon monoxide reading dropped to 3 ppm but rose to 14 ppm after smoking two cannabis cigarettes the night before her third appointment. This upset her very much and proved a far more powerful argument that smoking cannabis did effect her health than any words could. Anne resolved not to smoke cannabis again and her carbon monoxide reading returned to 3 ppm for the remainder of the therapy. Anne was often strongly tempted to smoke, particularly during the first four weeks. She avoided relapse by employing the same strategy as she had with her drinking; she increased her time spent in activities where smoking was not permitted. As her confidence increased her periods of anxiety became fewer and less acute.

Ending therapy

This patient cooperated fully in her therapy and in her fourth session decided that she had accomplished what she set out to achieve. This follows the BST premise of holding the number of sessions that the patient finds useful, not one more and not one less. The total time spent was a little under four hours and although Anne still described herself as a rather anxious person, she no longer felt disabled by stress. At six month follow up she was still not smoking and due to have her operation the next month. The CPN was no longer visiting and her number of consultations with her GP had halved.

Conclusion

Working in this way encourages professionals to consider the balance of time which we spend in discussing the past, the present and the future. The techniques of scaling and the use of the miracle question help the therapist and the patient move on from problem exploration. Problem focused thinking encourages the view that the patient is sick or inadequate and discourages the development of coping strategies. Solution focused thinking encourages awareness of how therapy is constructed, in particular of how language can determine the length of therapy or make problems appear solvable or unsolvable.

References

Alcoholics Anonymous (1983) *Twelve Steps and Twelve Traditions*. Alcoholics Anonymous World Services, New York.

Barret-Kruse, C. (1994) Brief counselling: a user's guide for traditionally trained counsellors. *International Journal for the Advancement of Counselling* **17**, 109–115.

Garfield, S.L. & Bergin, A.E., eds (1994) *Handbook of Psychotherapy and Behavior Change*, 4th edn. John Wiley & Sons, New York.

Hoyt, M.F. (1994) *Constructive Therapies*. Guilford Press, New York.

Marlatt, G. & Gordon, J. (1985) *Relapse Prevention*. Guilford Press, New York.

Miller, S.D. & Berg, I.K. (1995) *The Miracle Method*. W W Norton, New York.

Miller, S.D., Hubble, M.A. & Duncan, B.L., eds (1996) *Handbook of Solution Focused Brief Therapy*. Jossey-Bass, San Francisco.

Miller, W.R. & Rollnick, S. (1991) *Motivational Interviewing: Preparing People to Change. Addictive Behaviour*. Guilford Press, New York.

O'Connell, B. (1998) *Solution Focused Therapy*. Sage Publications, London.

Prochaska, J.O. & Di Clemente, C.C. (1986) Towards a comprehensive model of change. In: W. R. Miller & N. Heather (eds) *Treating Addictive Behaviours: Process of Change*. Plenum Press, New York.

de Shazer, S. (1994) *Words Were Originally Magic*. W W Norton, New York.

Silagy, C., Mant, D. & Fowler, G. (1998) *Nicotine Replacement Therapy for Smoking Cessation* (Cochrane review) ab000146-20012. In: The Cochrane Library Issue, 2 Oxford: Update Software.

13: Assessing Health and Social Needs and Develop Appropriate Services: A Public Health Perspective

Salman Rawaf

Introduction

The last few years in Britain have seen a political discovery and perhaps a wake up call on a subject everyone was willing to talk about but knew little of. Dual diagnosis is an elusive medical term to describe in a 'limited' way the coexistence of the two conditions of substance misuse (drugs and/or alcohol) and mental illness at the same time in one person (i.e. comorbidity). Both conditions are usually severe enough to warrant an intervention. The literature is littered with debate among generalist and specialist psychiatrists on the existence of such a relationship and its causes, the magnitude of the problem and above all who should be responsible for the care of these patients and how. In the midst of it all, there are patients who were either marginalised, or received in part inadequate care. This chapter addresses the population rather than the clinical dimension of the problem, as regards definition, magnitude, patients' needs, as well as service delivery, research agenda and future planning.

A problem of definition

Dual diagnosis is a term, which was first used by mental health professionals in the USA in the 1980s to describe the existence during the first diagnosis in the same individual at the same time of more than one medical condition. Although there is no clear agreement about what constitutes dual diagnosis, the term, however, is most often used to describe the coexistence (comorbidity) of mental health problems and substance misuse in the same individual. Such coexistence of two diagnoses raises many questions. What happens if a mentally ill person who misuses drugs or alcohol also has personality disorder? What will be the diagnosis if in addition to these two conditions the person suffers from acute or chronic physical problems? Does substance misuse lead to mental illness and vice versa? How long does it take before the two conditions are diagnosed in coexistence?

In the middle of this confusion, many professionals have expressed con-

cern about the social needs of people with coexisting problems. The terminology therefore has changed to 'complex needs' in an attempt to move
away from a solely medicalised definition of 'what are invariably complex
social problems that require a more holistic joined up approach if they are to
be tackled successfully' (Phillips & Labrow 1998).

Magnitude of the problem of dual diagnosis

In applying the definition above, in its strictest term, and without raising the
issue of whether the substance misuse leads to mental health problems and
vice versa, there is strong evidence that the prevalence of such coexistence is
much higher than identified and reported before. Figures of 30–50% of people with mental health problems who had current problematic drug and or
alcohol use, with an odds ratio of 4 for schizophrenia and 8 for bipolar affective disorders were reported from studies in the USA (Regier *et al.* 1990;
Khalsa *et al.* 1991). In the UK, the National Treatment Outcome Research
Study (NTORS) has found that around 10% of substance misuse patients had
had a history of psychiatric admission during the previous two years (Gossop
et al. 1998). Most recently Wright *et al.* (2000) reported a prevalence of
33% comorbidity of substance misuse and mental illness in a suburban
area. Prevalence is reported to be higher in urban compared with rural areas
(Menezes *et al.* 1996; Mueser *et al.* 2001). Comorbidity is associated with
young people, violence, severe symptoms and poor prognosis. Although comorbidity is associated with males, women tend to experience more severe
environmental, health, social and economic consequences and require more
costly care (Baker 2001). The public health risks associated with dual diagnosis in women are physical and sexual abuse, violence, HIV infection and
child welfare.

It is important to highlight the methodological limitations of these studies and lack of reliable population studies. Any estimate or prevalence for the
purpose of assessing the complex health and social needs of these patients
and thus planning and setting services to meet such needs should be treated
with caution. Such an exercise is complicated by the lack of any meaningful
outcome data.

Assessing health and social needs

Comprehensive health and social needs assessment is an essential starting
point for the development of any intervention strategy, service development
or health improvement programme for people with coexisting mental
health problems and substance misuse. Rawaf and Marshall (1999) have developed 10 practical steps for assessing health and social needs of drug misusers. A summary of these steps, which combine both the quantitative and
the qualitative approaches for health and social needs assessment is given in
Fig. 13.1 and they will now be examined in more detail.

As regards Step One, it is important to remember that while assessing the

Step one:	Understand your population size, structure, dynamic
	Segment your population
	↓
Step two:	Identify the incidence and prevalence of the condition/problem
	Use published local/national/international figures
	↓
Step three:	Calculate the expected number of cases (total, age groups, gender, etc.) Apply step 2 to step 1
	↓
Step four:	Measure service utilisation [health, social, housing, etc.] (self help, primary care, secondary care, specialist service)
	↓
Step five:	Calculate unmet needs Step 3 minus step 4
	↓
Step six:	Assess effectiveness of intervention(s) (EBM)
	↓
Step seven:	Seek population's views (experience, expectations)
	↓
Step eight:	Assess professionals' views [especially local one] (clinical practice, feasibility, barriers, etc.)
	↓
Step nine:	Define priorities [take into account current and new resources]
	↓
Step ten:	Advice on intervention(s)/ Health care programme(s)/ **Strategy**

Rawaf & Marshall, 1999.

Fig. 13.1 Ten steps of health needs assessment

population under surviellance, you need to take into account those who are in mental hospitals and prisons based within your locality or serving your population.

Steps Two and Three involve the initial calculation of the incidence/ prevalence of the problem under review, and a likely projection of these within the local population. As mentioned above the lack of reliable population prevalence studies may cause difficulties in obtaining reliable estimates of the number of the people who require the evidence based intervention and the support. It is advisable to work as a starting point with the low prevalence figures available and review it once services are developed. Base your review on both utilisation of services and effectiveness of interventions.

Steps Four and Five measure service usage to arrive at a calculation of unmet needs in the population. There is clear evidence that dually diagnosed patients are falling through the gaps between mental health services and substance misuse services. In the UK there are no defined services for the assessment, treatment and support of such patients, who have complex and diverse needs. Routine data on service utilisation by this group of patients are therefore scant.

Efficacy of intervention is estimated in Step Six. Evidence is emerging that effective dual diagnosis programmes must combine mental health and substance misuse interventions to best meet the complex needs of patients with comorbid disorders (Drake *et al.* 2001). A three-year randomised trial suggests that direct family support may help people with dual diagnosis to reduce or eliminate their substance use (Clark 2001). There are many arguments for and against specialist services for these groups of patients. However, further research is needed on the effective interventions and the modalities of service delivery.

Owing to the complexity and diversity of their needs it is essential to seek the views of these patients on the type of services, methods of delivery and the priorities to deal with them effectively (Step Seven). The literature provides little or no evidence of experience and expectations of these patients.

Having gathered the views of the service users, Step Eight is to do the same for the professional service providers. At the time of writing, at least in the UK, there is currently no agreement among various mental health professionals about what constitutes dual diagnosis, who should lead in assessing and treating these patients and how the services should be delivered. Their local views are therefore an essential step to define the services required.

From the information collated, priorities must now be set (Step Nine). Services needed for these patients are complex and some elements of it are costly. Any new service development needs to be addressed within the competing priorities. Shifting resources from existing services, re-engineering services and disinvestment in ineffective or redundant services should be considered as part of the process of defining priorities.

Step Ten is to mould an overall strategic plan which embraces all the content of the first nine steps. Any emerging recommendations and plans need to be feasible, practical and affordable. Otherwise the carefully formulated strategy will be condemned to finish on the shelf, collecting dust.

Intervention strategies

The complex natures of substance misuse and mental health, each in its own right and in coexistence, means that no single intervention strategy has yet been singled out as effective in reducing the burden of the condition at individual or community level.

Any strategy to deal with the existence of dual diagnosis/comorbidity should aim to:

- reduce or eliminate the substance misuse
- manage and change the psychiatric symptoms.

Primary prevention

Drugs can cause, exacerbate and or precipitate mental illness. Prevention of substance misuse therefore will certainly help to reduce the overall burden of comorbidities in the community. A comprehensive public health approach based on discouraging new recruits, reaching those not in touch with any service, and harm reduction to tackle the diverse aspects of drug use and misuse is more promising (Rawaf 1998).

Primary prevention could also aim at preventing, for example, patients with mental health problems from abusing drugs and or alcohol. Early recognition of mental illness including 'common' disorders (for example depression and anxiety), is therefore essential. The role of primary health care teams is crucial in this area. Screening for depression in primary care is one of many strategies to identify problems at an early stage. Reducing the severity of mental illness through early diagnosis and treatment, support and care plan may reduce or eliminate reliance on substance misuse among these patients. Prison diversion programmes may reduce the high risk of drug uses and misuse within the prison.

Developing appropriate services

Patients diagnosed as 'dual' are falling through the gaps between mental health services on the one hand and specialist substance misuse services on the other hand. This is the result of the rigidity of professional boundaries in health care delivery and treatment ideologies and an undesirable by-product of medical subspecialisation. Evidence from literature and local services indicates that patients with a dual diagnosis label have shown little or no contact with services, early disengagement, poor or non-compliance with treatment and medication and increased levels of suicide thoughts, attempts and deaths (Pristach & Smith 1990; Ridgely *et al.* 1990; Kessler *et al.* 1996; Department of Health 1999)

Due to the multiple problems and chaotic lifestyle patients with comorbidity require proper assessment and detailed plans for their treatment and care. The present difficulty with this is the lack of appropriate and tested models to deal with these cases. There are many proposed models for consecutive, parallel and integrated treatment, but none has been fully researched and its outcomes measured.

A new integrated approach

Building on local experience and the difficulties we encountered in providing an acceptable model for patients with possible diagnosis of comorbidity, an integrated care pathway as shown in Fig. 13.2 has been introduced and funded as a pilot within three Community Mental Health Teams, one in each of the Boroughs of Merton, Sutton and Wandsworth, in southern England. The intention is to provide an operational interface between primary health care services and community mental health teams, and access to specialist and ancillary services as required for each patient.

The work of the Primary Care Team includes:

- the bulk of the prevention of substance misuse (working closely with addiction prevention practitioners);
- promotion of mental health;
- early diagnosis and early intervention;

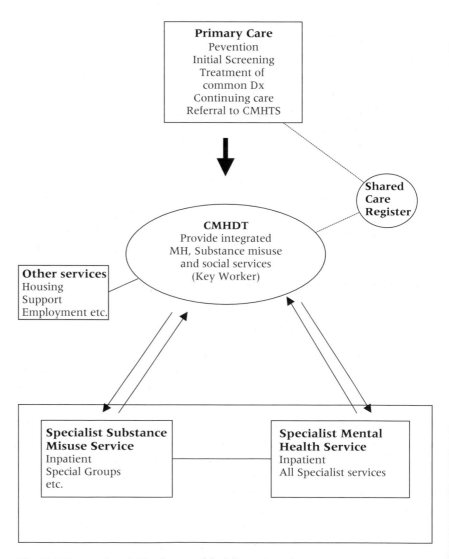

Fig. 13.2 Proposed model for the care of dual diagnosis patients

- referral to the CMHT;
- continuing the care of these patients and their carers (as part of the shared care approach);
- crisis management and referral as necessary;
- coordination with the designated key worker and general health of the patients; and maintaining the shared care register jointly with the CMHT (Strathdee *et al.* 1999).

Community Mental Health Teams involved in the scheme will see their role broadened through the incorporation of their expertise in dealing with substance misuse and provision of social services. Their functions will include:
- the systematic assessment of health and social needs of each patient and his or her carer;
- development of an integrated care plan (ICPA) with a designated key worker assigned to each patient;
- assertive community treatment for those who need it (Strathdee *et al.* 1999);
- regular review of patients' progress in collaboration with the primary care team (shared care approach); and
- referral to specialist services (mental health or substance misuse), and jointly maintaining the shared care register.

Due to the complexity of the multiple problems encountered by these patients, some of them need services in either specialised mental health or substance misuse units or both. Such referrals are the remit of the CMHTs, who are also responsible for access to other services from various sources. For example, the homeless need shelter and subsequently permanent accommodation, employment and other services. Women with comorbidity may need protection from abuse and childcare services. Those with dual diagnosis who are in prison (the scheme does not extend to cover serious crimes) may benefit from a prison diversion programme (Mueser *et al.* 2001).

A reflection on current services

Current studies and commissioning experience at local level indicate that pa tients with comorbidity of substance misuse and mental health are not accessing available facilities because of the reasons mentioned above. A radical look at both mental health and substance misuse services is needed to address this inequality in health care provision. The model outline above will raise many questions about the current roles of the Community Mental Health Team and the way such a role should be expanded and supported with the necessary resources and training (for example a Community Mental Health and Drug Team). Many other questions could also be raised in relation to the future of substance misuse services. What would be the role of the Community Drug Teams, once the CMHDTs are undertaking their new expanded role? What will be the relationship between the specialist substance misuse services and the CMHDTs and the specialist mental health services? It is no longer acceptable to use comorbidity as an excuse to 'buck pass' these patients and allow them to fall between services.

Conclusion: a challenging research agenda

The high prevalence of the coexistence of mental health and substance misuse emerging as a public health problem requires urgent attention. These groups of patients have complex needs associated with multiple problems and chaotic lifestyle. Current health and social care facilities are not accessible due to many professional and organisational barriers. Solutions are possible through re-engineering of the services, investment and training to create robust models of service delivery sensitive to the needs of these patients and their carers.

For health authorities, primary care groups and services providers the first step is to assess this group's health and social needs and develop the strategies to meet such needs. For practitioners and the research community this is a rich field to invest some scientific resources to provide some answers to the questions raised above.

There is very little research evidence from the UK on the aetiology of dual diagnosis, or the prevention of one or both elements of it, the most effective intervention models, methods of service delivery, patients' and carers' views and perception and measures of outcome. The political wake up call we are receiving may be an opportunity for professionals to address the needs of these patients.

References

Baker, D.R. (2001) Substance abuse and mental illness: unaddressed public health issues for women. *Journal of the American Medical Women's Association* **56**, 27–28.

Clark, R.E. (2001) Family support and substance use outcomes for persons with mental illness and substance use disorders. *Schizophrenia Bulletin* **27**, 93–101.

Department of Health (1999) *Safer Services: National Inquiry into Suicide and Homicide by People with Mental Illness*. Department of Health, London.

Drake, R.E., Essock, S.M., Shanner, A. *et al.* (2001) Implementing dual diagnosis services for clients with severe mental illness. *Psychiatric Services* **52**, 469–476.

Gossop, M., Marsden, J. & Steward, D. (1998) *NTORS at one year: The National Treatment and Outcome Research Study*. Department of Health, London.

Kessler, R.C., Nelson, C. & McGonagle, K. (1996) The epidemiology of co-occurring addictive and mental disorders. Implications for prevention and service utilisation. *American Journal of Orthopsychiatry* **66**, 17–31.

Khalsa, H.K., Shanner, A., Anglin, M.D. *et al.* (1991) Prevalence of substance abuse in a psychiatric evaluation unit. *Drug and Alcohol Dependence* **28** (2), 15–18.

Menezes, P. R., Johnson, S., Thornicroft, G. *et al.* (1996) Drug and alcohol problems among individuals with severe mental illness in south London. *British Journal of Psychiatry* **168,** 612–619.

Mueser, K.T., Bond, G.R. & Drake, R.E. (2001) Community-based treatment of schizophrenia and other severe mental disorders. *Medscape Mental Health* **6** (1), 1–10.

Phillips, P. & Labrow, J. (1998) *Dual Diagnosis*. Mind, London.

Pristach, C.A. & Smith, C.M. (1990) Medication compliance and substance abuse among psychiatric patients. *Hospital Community Psychiatry* **41**, 1345–1348.

Rawaf, S. (1998) Public health and addiction: prevention. *Current Opinion in Psychiatry* **11**, 1273–1278.

Rawaf, S. & Marshall, F. (1999) Drug misuse: the ten steps for needs assessment. *Public Health Medicine* **1**, 21–26.

Regier, D.A., Farmer, M.E., Rae, D.S. *et al.* (1990) Comorbidity of mental disorders with alcohol and other drug abuse. Results from the Epidemiological Catchment Area (ECA) study. *Journal of the American Medical Association* **264**, 2511–2518.

Ridgely, M.S., Goldman, H.H. & Willenbring, M. (1990) Barriers to the care of persons with dual diagnosis: organisational and financial issues. *Schizophrenia Bulletin* **16**, 123–132.

Strathdee, G., Jenkins, R., Carr, S. & Rawaf, S. (1999) Equity in mental health: what should public health practitioners do? *Public Health Medicine* **2**, 61–67.

Wright, S., Gournay, K., Glorney, E. & Thornicroft, G. (2000) Dual diagnosis in the suburbs: prevalence, need and in-patient service use. *Social Psychiatry and Psychiatric Epidemiology* **35**, 297–304.

14: Development of a Community Based Model of Service Provision for Dual Diagnosis Patients

Alison Lowe

Background

Elsewhere in this book the definitions and epidemiology of dual diagnosis will have been well described. From mid 1998 as a consultant psychiatrist I have been the lead clinician involved in a mental health led initiative to develop a community based dual diagnosis service in the multi-ethnic urban setting of the London Borough of Haringey, England. Many people collaborated with this project and continue to help it along its way and through some difficult patches. It has needed considerable innovation as there is no model to copy in the United Kingdom (UK) and we have had to develop it from first principles of care for addictions and mental health problems. In this chapter the principles behind the service that now functions in Haringey will be presented and some of the problems encountered and the solutions will be highlighted.

Problems to consider

Need for a local solution

It is acknowledged that the specific elements of a community based service have to be local. This needs to reflect not only the local treatment services that are in place in the voluntary and statutory sectors but also whatever information exists about the scope and scale of dual diagnosis in the area. In terms of mental health profile the borough of Haringey is an area of London with a high bed occupancy rate for psychiatry, a diverse ethnic mix and a large proportion of refugees (OPCS 1991). Mental health care is focused around individuals with major morbidity and the new dual diagnosis service developed to parallel this. In the context of the development of the Haringey service, dual diagnosis is defined as 'The cooccurrence of serious mental illness and the suspicion of a substance misuse problem'. This reflects some uncertainty around the diagnosis of substance misuse problems. With respect to substance misuse in Haringey, there was an awareness that after alcohol, 'crack' cocaine is probably the most commonly misused drug and we did not expect very much heroin use in the dual diagnosis population. This meant for example, that there was no need for substitute prescribing for opiate abuse to constitute a major part of the new service.

The evidence base and the health care system

A literature search will produce a lot of information from the USA with complex acronyms and references to 'programs'. The UK health care system is anchored in general practice and promises to supply free care at point of entry. In the UK, patients are not used to the idea of belonging to a programme or to the idea that entry to a programme would then provide funding for this 'episode' of care. The dual diagnosis programme described by Drake *et al.* (1993) that is able to take patients in, provide all their health care needs and hold onto them for up to five years, is not a viable option in resource terms or in context of current health care planning.

The mental health services are responding to the Government document *The National Service Framework*, addiction is functioning under Drug Action Team templates and the National Strategy for Alcohol is not yet published. Within these frameworks patients who have major mental health problems and substance misuse problems still need treatment. The approach chosen was to bridge the gaps not by another free-standing service but by trying to develop a responsive, flexible service to help patients access care in networks that already exist. The service works as an adjunct to the care the patient already has and is not a substitute for other services remaining or becoming involved.

Two different views

Another difficult area to consider is the difference in philosophies between traditional addiction services and mental health provision. In addiction services the patient (more usually called client) is responsible for their own behaviour and can leave an interview or walk out of a residential rehabilitation setting if they so wish. In a mental health context, if a practitioner is concerned (for example about the nature and severity of psychotic symptoms) common law or statutory legislation may be used to stop a patient leaving. Indeed patients with a wide range of conditions from anorexia to schizophrenia may be admitted against their wishes for assessment and treatment under the Mental Health Act if they are found to be at sufficient risk. Admission for treatment for addiction alone is specifically excluded from the current act (Mental Health Act 1983). As a general principle, the mental health practitioner is more likely to assume a responsibility for a patient and intervene than an addictions worker is. The addiction field has embraced motivational interviewing as described by Miller and Rollnick (1991). The component of our role is about persuading and empowering patients to make changes against the apparent odds. The distance between the differing philosophical stances may be decreasing as treatment options in the UK now are increasingly being linked to the criminal justice system. The introduction of Drug Treatment and Testing Orders remains a controversial area but has introduced the idea of compulsion into treatment for drug (but not alcohol) problems. Mental health is using motivational interviewing to help with compliance and skills in the fields are becoming more complementary and closely aligned.

Stigma and prejudice

It became apparent talking about the patients with substance misuse problems and a major mental illness that certain workers find them very difficult even to talk about. In part this reflects a sense of not having the skills in all areas and also an underlying sense of 'what do I do with this information if I collect it?' There is a feeling of 'better leave it alone' linked to a sense of hopelessness and therapeutic pessimism. This is fuelled by ignorance of treatment options and also a sense that the dual diagnosis itself may lead to exclusion. If a mental health hostel knows an individual is using crack cocaine it will be less likely to accept them. Prejudice and stigma exist around both mental health and addiction. The issue of addiction invoking moral judgements, particularly around the way that an individual funds a drug habit and whether they can then 'benefit from mental health care' is one that arises in some staff groups. On the other hand, some individuals with a substance use problem (and some of the staff working with them) do not want to be seen as having any links to 'madness' or be linked with psychiatry. The final prejudice encountered is a concern that resources might be diverted away from established services in both fields to support these exceptional patients. In one way it seems appropriate that funding should follow the individuals with great need but this does not make for easy working conditions with colleagues and the injection of 'new' funding to this project was felt to be essential.

Expectations and demand

The epidemiology of dual diagnosis tells us that 60% of our psychiatric patients may be using either drugs or alcohol (Menezes *et al.* 1996) and this may be affecting their mental health. This provides a huge potential demand, before including individuals who may have significant mental health difficulties and are only in contact with an addiction team.

In a health care and political climate where outcomes are being measured there is a sense of not wanting to be burdened with these patients. It would seem obvious that a caseload biased towards dual diagnosis or comorbidity does not tend to improve the outcome statistics. This in turn leads to a desire to transfer the patients off caseload and into any new dual diagnosis service that may be established. This risks swamping the new service with sheer numbers of patients, blocking the treatment slots and producing a waiting list. There is also the risk of the service becoming a dumping ground for (these are my quotes) 'the worst of the worst'. These are the difficult and dangerous psychiatric patients who misuse alcohol and other illegal drugs, which in turn introduce more disinhibited and illegal behaviours. The cycle continues as their psychiatric mental state deteriorates and there is the fear of serious harm to themselves or others. This is a difficult and unreliable treatment paradigm, which is not a pleasant prospect for the new embryo team and may be a factor in recruitment. Given these heavy demands how does the dual diagnosis service decide whom it will see and work with? This has to be an issue of boundaries, referral criteria, and a model of service intervention, all of which had to be developed on a local basis in Haringey. The next section describes the different stages of establishing the project there.

The Haringey model dual diagnosis service

Establishing a steering group

There are a wide variety of individuals and organisations that wished to contribute to the discussion around this issue and an open inclusive forum was our aim. In practical terms this had to be supported and chaired and individuals of sufficient status in their organisations to commit to and make decisions were needed. The membership of the Haringey Dual Diagnosis steering group is given in Table 14.1.

The function of the group differed through the initial phase of information gathering, development and submission of the bid and the early days of the service development. At times there were conflicts over what was seen as possible or desirable. The overwhelming need for a service was seen as coming from mental health, the trust supported the steering group and the bid was led from mental health, with the writer involved as a consultant psychiatrist. The service is now located there (see later), but has good links to substance misuse and other services.

Questions to ask

Initially the steering group needed to ask a series of questions.
Is there a need? How much do we know about the patient group locally?
What services do we have locally?
What resources do we have?
Who do we need to talk to?
What fits in locally?

These questions led to a series of things that needed to be done:

(1) *Local needs assessment*: This comprised the summation of what information we already had about the size and nature of the dual diagnosis in the area. It included surveys done by the drug service, an outreach worker in mental health, information from the alcohol agency and mental health statistics. Following this a more detailed survey was commissioned.

181

Table 14.1 Dual diagnosis steering group

The following were included from the Trust
Consultant Psychiatrist Mental Health and Addiction Services
Team Leader Dual Diagnosis Service (once appointed)
Service Manager   Mental Health Trust
Senior Manager   Child & Adolescent Services
Manager Drug Treatment Service
Chief Executive St Ann's Hospital
Senior Practitioner Mental Health Outreach Haringey
Senior Practitioner Ethnic Outreach Project Haringey
General Manager

From the Health Authority
Finance Director Mental Health & Addiction Services. Haringey Health
                                   Authority
DAT Coordinator Health Authority

From Social Services
Senior Manager in Haringey Social Services, special responsibility for housing
Director Mental Health Services adjacent borough

Other addiction services
Outreach Worker   Adjacent Borough Drug and Alcohol Service
Manager   Adjacent Borough Drug and Alcohol Service
Director Voluntary Sector Agency for alcohol treatment covering Haringey and
adjacent borough

From collaborating academic institutions (who did initial needs assessment)
Clinical Nurse specialist
Clinical Psychologist

Representatives from local community police also attended

(2) *Mapping exercise of resources and networks*: This was done in principle (see Fig. 14.1) and then in practice on the two maps shown. They include the obvious as well as broader links to probation, maternity care, etc. This exercise shows how complex a network these patients may need to be in contact with.

(3) *What would 'fit' locally*: This is the process of deciding what will work locally, putting in a bid and planning the service.

History/needs assessment

On the understanding that a free-standing service would not be chosen and that recruitment woud consist of 'in' patients of several years, a model appropriate to the needs of the local population would be developed. This type of service would function well in the British system with its strong primary health care history and locality provided mental health and addiction teams. There was also an awareness that some patients had excellent links for example into mental health but no contact with any addiction service, despite having major drug or alcohol problems. The aim was to design a service that was flexible and able to provide for or obtain rapid access for an individual

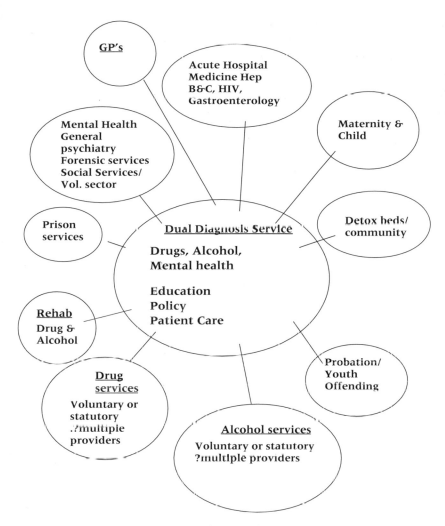

Fig. 14.1 Map of service connections in principle. © ALL-2001

into the clinical care they might need at that moment. This may range from an assessment and action on a depressed mental state or information on 'crack' cocaine. It was important that individuals from the long standing support structures that are around these patients (e.g. the community mental health nurse from the CMHT or the supportive GP) would not be excluded. In the long term this service seeks to educate those caring for these patients and to empower the patients themselves so that an integration of care to match a patient's assessed problems can be achieved.

Thus the working group set up in Haringey had an ambitious remit. Within the resource limitations, the aims were not only to provide a clinical service but also to educate, teach about and research what was happening, as well as change the attitude of individuals and the climate of the organisations the patients encountered.

With local consultation under way and set within the National Health

Service framework, a liaison style adjunctive team to bridge gaps in patient care without removing patients from support that is present was established. The service has different arms, one for direct patient care, one for educating, researching and teaching and one for what is labelled organisational issues. The way the service is set up is a result of local solutions to the awareness of the difficulties of this population and their enormous needs as well as the very high expectations set externally. The Haringey Dual Diagnosis team does not see patients in isolation. They retain their links into either an addiction team or a Community Mental Health service.

The nature of the service

Staffing

The service is led by a consultant psychiatrist and when setting up we endeavoured to make the grades of other staff as high as possible (see Table 14.2). This is to reflect the fact that it was important that the staff had to be already able in one interview to deal with whatever psychiatric symptoms or addictions problem that was being presented (or trainable to achieve this). The grading of jobs as highly as possible was instituted to overcome possible recruitment problems (why should anyone come and deal with such a population perceived as difficult with no extra status or pay?).

Referral criteria

This is an issue which would seem to be fairly straightforward but can become complex. These criteria are what set the boundaries for the team, and protect the new service from becoming swamped by sheer weight of referrals. The criteria used in Haringey are shown in Table 14.3. The key criteria for our service are a diagnosis of mental illness and problems with substance misuse and residence in (or collection of benefits from) the London Borough

Table 14.2 Staff complement Haringey dual service

Consultant Psychiatrist	1	0.5WTE
Clinical Assistant	1 (unfilled)	0.5WTE
Team Leader	1H Grade	1WTE
CPN	2G Grade	2WTE
Senior Practitioner Outreach	1 A & C 7	1WTE
Dual Diagnosis Worker	1 A & C 6	1WTE
Outreach Worker	1 A & C 5	1WTE
Senior Administrator	1 A & C 5	1WTE
Medical Secretary	1 A & C 4	0.5WTE
Secretary	1 A & C 3	0.5WTE
Psychologist	(unfilled)	1WTE
Research Psychologist		1WTE (1 year contract)

Table 14.3 Referral criteria (taken from our information leaflets)

- All referrals must be aged between 18 and 65 years
- All referred patients must have a diagnosed mental health problem, and a substance use problem
- Individuals with a diagnosis of Personality Disorder can be referred to this service
- All referrals must live within the catchment area of Haringey Healthcare NHS Trust (including Edmonton)
- All referrals must be discussed with the patient, and the patient must agree to the referral

(Referral forms must be signed by a Consultant Psychiatrist and either a Sector Manager or Ward Manager.)

When we are unable to accept referrals:
- Patients who are outside the ages of 18 and 65 years
- Where there is a learning disability
- Where the patient has a primary physical diagnosis and a substance use problem
- Where there has been no risk assessment completed on the patient
- Where the referral form has not been fully completed
- We are not able to accept self-referrals
- We are not able to accept referrals directly from General Practitioners

of Haringey. We then also accept 'suspicion of mental illness' in referrals from agencies in addiction that do not have medically trained psychiatric cover. We do not exclude any particular group of substance misusers (we have heard of some teams excluding alcohol misusers if that is the sole drug) nor do we exclude those patients with a diagnosis of personality disorder. The geographical issues may not be clear in an area, as for example our Mental Health Trust extends onto an adjacent borough by a population block of about 100 000 people. Understandably my general psychiatry colleagues want us to cover their wards, but we have to cooperate with a different addictions team to those relating to the rest of the borough.

The dual diagnosis team does not take referrals from GPs or directly from agencies outside of the borough of Haringey (including forensic services and prison) in part due to resource implications but also to keep the links to local services. As to when people moving in become 'local' we follow the guidance used by the Mental Health Trust. The criteria for age are those of adult mental health (16–65) which leads to our colleagues in the Elderly Mental Ill Service complaining of their exclusion. There was also an insistance that the patient is aware of the referral and that the referral form is signed by a consultant, ward manager, team leader or sector manager. This provides some boundary protection and means that my consultant colleagues are aware of who they have referred. If the patient is from mental health a current Risk Assessment form is required. The following patients were excluded (after many discussions): patients with organic brain syndromes and those with severe learning difficulties. It was felt that this group of patients would have problems with the psychological interventions that would be used (particularly those focused around addiction).

Physical location

There is always an issue with a new service as to where it is located physically. Rooms to see patients, clinical space for examinations, minor procedures, e.g. wound dressings as well as larger rooms for meetings and groups, significant administrative space, and office space for staff are needed. The need for security is substantial but also the space needs to feel welcoming and humanising for patients and staff alike.

The current location of the service is in well appointed refurbished accommodation in the Mental Health Trust premises on a multi use hospital site. The quality of the refurbishment has attracted covetous glances and evoked stigmatising and prejudicial comments. The staff still do a significant amount of work away from the unit, seeing patients in the wards at the mental health or addiction team premises or on home visits.

Management funding and service organisation

This issue parallels exactly the problems of dual diagnosis. The steering group should engage with and have wide membership from both voluntary and statutory agencies, addictions and mental health, hospital, community, police probation, etc. Once discussions have taken place someone has to take responsibility and act to take a project forward. Even the preparation of a bid will involve meetings, paper work, coffee to be ordered, etc. The question of who this falls to, and if you are successful in bidding, who will manage the service, appoint staff and help with premises has to be addressed. The balance of leadership is an issue that needs to be decided locally. In Haringey the greatest pressure for the Dual Diagnosis Service came from the mental health service and our initial senior management was from the Child and Adult Community Services sector. A local solution is needed but clarity and consistency as well as a sense of humour are essential ingredients to this style of cross boundary working.

Risk assessment and management

This group of patients may be seen as difficult to assess and demanding to work with. Mental health services have been inundated with statutory requirements for the Care Plan Approach (CPA) and risk assessments. The paperwork attached varies in local areas, but having been developed from the mental health perspective usually all substance misuse is marked together as being high risk. There was little attempt to differentiate patterns of substance use and highlight more chaotic periods, when a clinical assessment by someone with addiction experience points to patients running higher risks. Dual diagnosis patients may have risk assessments already in place or the service may need to initiate it. The challenge is to adapt risk assessment tools so they pick up the risk in addictive behaviour as well as the mental health risks. The management of clinical risk is beyond the scope of this chapter. Essentially it is rooted in careful assessment, high quality clinical care based in practice and protocol, multidisciplinary working and information sharing. This in turn requires a cross boundary confidentiality policy with other parts of the health service, social services and some of the voluntary sector that we are fortunate to have in place in Haringey. When a service is being set up there are other risks to be assessed. The usual health and safety items need considering as well as the security of premises and staffing levels. Safety issues around home visiting and outreach work need to be thought through and may have resource implications (e.g. mobile phones for staff and a reliable phone back system to cover 'risky' visits). There may be local protocols already in place for this particularly in mental health, which can be adapted.

What does the service do?

Direct patient care and services offered

Assessment

It became apparent that a major part of the role of the team is to provide an accurate and detailed multidisciplinary assessment which may take more than one appointment. The inclusion of time lines and standardised assessment tools (borrowed from both mental health and addiction even though they have not been formally tested in this group) all aid the aim of a clear summary of the current situation and background. There is the recognition that in the UK hospitals code diagnosis in ICD 10 but find that at assessment DSM-IV may be a more helpful tool. All referrals are allocated at the weekly multidisciplinary team meeting and assessments fed back the week of their completion. A written summary of the assessment is sent to the referrer with a management plan attached. (Note, high levels of written communications are essential to this team, needing significant levels of administrative support telephone lines and computer access.

Multiple copies of letters from the consultant referrer, GP, Community Mental Health Team at a different address to the consultant or hostel manager are common occurrences. Patients have to give consent for information sharing unless there is an issue of risk when confidentiality may be breached, but there are relatively few problems with this in practice.) Assessments follow a bio-psychosocial model and should include physical examination, routine blood tests and urine drug screening.

Shorter term interventions

The key to the model of service in Haringey is the issue of it bridging gaps between other services to provide appropriate and as far as possible evidence based treatment following the intensive diagnosis and assessment described

Table 14.4 What we offer (taken from our information leaflet)

Any intervention that is offered by this service is time limited. We usually work with individuals for 3–6 months.
Outreach services can work with individuals for up to 1 year.
- Comprehensive mental health and substance use assessments
- Joint assessments with other agencies
- Individualised case management and counselling approaches
- Substitute prescribing for certain patient groups
- Multidisciplinary approach
- Assertive outreach programme
- Medical and psychiatric health screening
- Education
- Research relation to dual diagnosis
- Advice and information
- Publication of The Rough Guide to Addictions for Mental Health Wards
- The Dual Diagnosis Professionals Forum

above. Whilst the evidence base for interventions in dual diagnosis is limited, the principles of interventions from psychiatry and addiction are followed. This requires a breadth of skills in the team from educational interventions to the obvious medical role of initiating medication such as antidepressants or methadone, to motivational interviewing, relapse prevention and psychotherapeutic skills as well as behavioural and social interventions such as liaison with housing and benefits agencies. There are other services that offer a specific intervention to the dually diagnosed patient (e.g. cognitive behavioural therapy) but when the service was set up there was a strong notion that the patients needed this flexibility and range within one location. Indeed whilst the treatment systems battle with issues around provision for dual diagnosis the patients generate clinical problems that cross the boundaries with ease.

The aim of the short-term intervention is to do a focused, time limited piece of work and then pass the patient onto one of the long-term agencies (possibly having helped their staff to work more easily with this individual). This should in theory keep a throughput with the team promoting a mix of caseload and helping to protect against burnout and a service that is clogged and has an impossible waiting list. The time limit on these interventions is supposed to be 12 weeks, but in reality patients may over run or be re-referred. Interventions offered are shown in Table 14.4.

Longer term assertive outreach

In conjunction with the assessment and short-term interventions the service has a limited number of places for ongoing assertive outreach. Currently 30 patients, some poly substance users, represent the more chronic psychiatric patients. They are taken on for a (renewable) period of one year. These patients tend to have more unstable psychiatric illness and are more likely to be admitted under the Mental Health Act than the group with short-term interventions. Their substance misuse tends to be multiple including alcohol and relatively few of them have needed substitute prescribing with methadone. The principles of the interventions with them tend to follow the evidence base from psychiatry needing to be flexible and intensive.

Services offered to families

In parallel with the short-term interventions, sessions for carers/family members, particularly around addiction education are offered.

Education, teaching and research

With the staff mix recruited, there is a significant amount of skill and expertise that can be shared both ways to addictions and mental health to the benefits of patients and staff. A series of seminars were provided for the staff and as part of the service evaluation a baseline about education and attitudes was established in order to evaluate the impact over time. The issues and pressures surrounding research vs. service provision will vary by location. In Haringey, this service is being evaluated and we are looking at family interventions. The main priority remains the provision of clinical service. All members of the team are involved in their own ongoing professional development, and attend and participate in conferences, guideline development, etc. Several staff are doing or have completed higher degrees and a supportive attitude to study is a good antidote to the stresses of working with this group of patients and their complex problems.

Organisational issues

As well as directly working with patients and staff there is a range of issues around organisation and policy that we have been involved in. These include:
* confidentiality policy/sharing of information
* drugs on ward policy (mental health)
* alcohol detoxification policy (mental health)
* 'Rough guide to addiction' on mental health wards.
The Dual Diagnosis Service has also been in the forums of the Drug Action Team and the Mental Health Planning Group, to try to keep the needs of these patients on the wider agenda.

References

Drake, R.E., Bartels, S.J., Teague, G.B., Noordsy, D.L. & Clarke, R.E. (1993) Treatment of substance abuse in severely mentally ill patients. *Journal of Nervous and Mental Disorders* **181**, 606–611.

Menezes, P.R., Johnson, S., Thornicroft, G. *et al.* (1996) Drug and alcohol problems among individuals with severe mental illness in South London. *British Journal of Psychiatry* **168**, 612–619.

Mental Health Act (1983) HMSO, London.

Miller, W.R. & Rollnick, S. (1991) Motivational interviewing. *Preparing People to Change Addictive Behaviour*. Guilford Press, New York.

OPCS (1991) Census data for London Borough of Haringey. *1993 Census*. HMSO, London.

15: A Model of Treatment for Dual Diagnosis (The Greenbank Model)

Daisy Saffer

Introduction

The management of patients with dual diagnosis poses serious problems for service providers. Patients with comorbidity problems are assessed by services either as drug users with minor mental health problems or as patients with severe mental health problems who happen to have a substance misuse problem. They are not seen as suffering from comorbidity as a specific problem and therefore deserving a planned and comprehensive response to their comorbidity. The comorbidity of psychiatric disorders and substance misuse disorders has greatly increased since the early 1980s. This rapid increase has meant service provision and clinical practice have lagged behind the demands for treatment. There is however, an increased interest in understanding why such a strong association between these disorders exists and research is advancing in the area rapidly. This advancement has now moved towards providing a better and more comprehensive management of these disorders.

The Greenbank Unit (established in 1967 as a regional alcohol rehabilitation unit) has in the last few years moved towards recognising that the majority of the patients referred to the unit have complex needs (dual or multiple diagnosable disorders) and are often suffering from recognised mental illness in addition to their addiction. In addition, 50–60% of patients referred to the unit are misusing at least one or more other psychoactive substances in addition to alcohol. The most common drugs are cannabis, benzodiazepine, heroin and cocaine. As a result of the prevalence of dual diagnosis, the unit has developed a specific and comprehensive treatment programme based on full assessment and treatment. The key aim is to ensure that comorbidity is recognised and addressed as a composite problem rather than a series of loosely connected health and behavioural issues. This results in the team being able to address all the issues underlying the disorders and providing effective interventions.

Greenbank Substance Recovery Centre is a National Health Service unit which provides treatment, supportive and rehabilitative service for patients recovering from alcohol/drug misuse and their families. Greenbank is a therapeutic community that offers multi-professional psychotherapeutic approaches to care and treatment of patients with complex needs. The services are based upon a range of psychotherapeutic treatment including detoxification treatment, rehabilitation and discharge to appropriate accommodation, follow-up facilities and crisis intervention.

It has facilities for 16 inpatients and 12 day patients who have a current primary problem with alcohol or other psychoactive substances and or psychiatric morbidities.

Programme design

The programme is designed in seven stages which are able to accommodate individual goal setting and is committed to deliver needs-led service. Table 15.1 provides an outline of the programme design.

Elements of the service

The 'Greenbank Model' (see Figs. 15.1, 15.2) offers a comprehensive integrated treatment programme based around four distinct stages:

(1) full and comprehensive assessment;

(2) detoxification;

(3) inpatient treatment programme—interim day programme; and

(4) after-care programme.

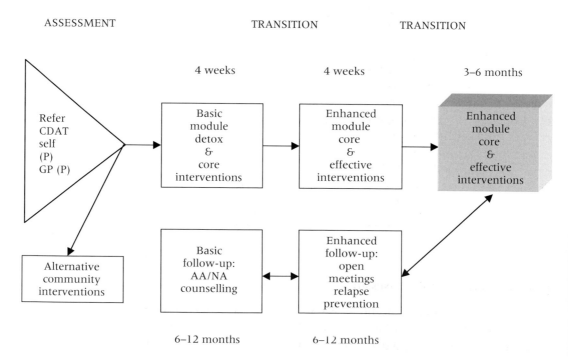

Fig. 15.1 Schematic view of new Greenbank modular treatment

Table 15.1 Greenbank substance misuse recovery centre programme design

Stages	Contents
Stage 1 (1 week)	Orientation to substance misuse problems Assessment process Education on associated problems Agreeing goals for treatment Agreeing a treatment plan Assessing motivation to change Appraise extent of problems Setting realistic objectives (admission to residential/ rehabilitation unit)

Stage 2 (2 weeks)	Orientation—unit/ground environment
	Assimilation into therapeutic group—entering in the
	    programme and keeping diary
	Client remains on the unit and within hospital grounds
	More active participation in group
	Client allowed off premises accompanied by senior group
	    member
	Client has formulation of alcohol/substance related problems
	    and therapeutic goals
	Involvement of significant others in the therapeutic community

Stage 3 (1 week)	Preparation of life story Presentation of life story Detailed review of the therapeutic goal to include relationships, emotional as well as behavioural changes Weekend leave with attainable and progressive therapeutic goal
Stage 4 (1 week)	Group leadership Developing coping strategies Attitude change Consolidate weekend leave
Stage 5 (1 week)	Reflection Set intermediate objectives Focus work Planning discharge
Stage 6 (1 week)	Evaluation of therapeutic process Focus work Discharge Set follow-up programme
Stage 7 (2 weeks)	Focus work Follow-up Target relevant issues revealed by discharge

Full and comprehensive assessment

Following a period of detoxification it is possible that individuals suffering from comorbidity can be identified by means of relatively straightforward assessment. It is acknowledged that most patients with a substance use problem might have psychiatric symptoms, these are usually relieved within two

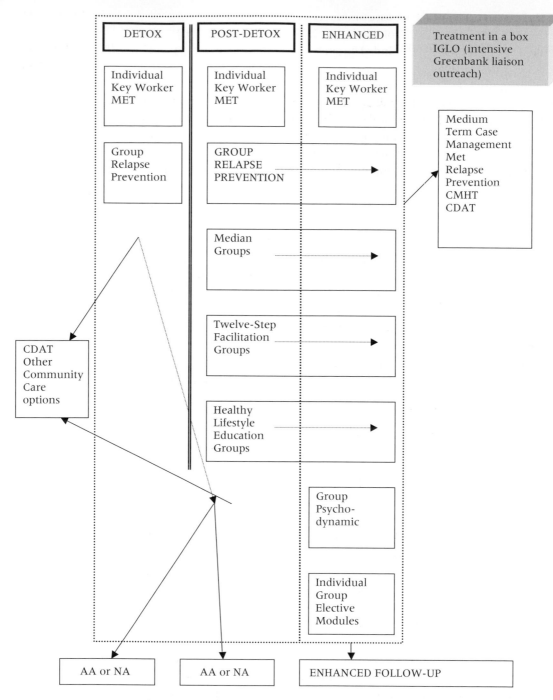

Fig. 15.2 Greenbank substance misuse recovery centre programme

to four weeks. Before their assessment is commenced the patients are required to be drug and alcohol free for a minimum of 24 h. This allows the patient to be alert and clear-minded enough to understand the concept and function of assessment.

The full assessment consists of:

(1) Full and comprehensive drug and alcohol history including preprescribed medication, features of dependency and signs and symptoms of withdrawal, in addition to comprehensive enquiries regarding complications (physical, psychological and social) of addiction.

(2) Comprehensive assessment of patients' mental status and establishing accurate psychiatric history, corroborated by general practitioners (GP), community mental health teams (CMHT) and other agencies involved in patients' care. Patients with stable mild and moderate psychiatric disorders are included in the programme. Those with more serious psychiatric disorders, especially florid psychoses, need a period of stabilisation before they are included in the programme. Caution must always be exercised in the interests of the patients, and alternative case management programmes are seen to be more relevant to a minority of patients with much more serious disorders where the possibility of patients fragmenting under the stress of the group intervention has to be considered.

(3) The establishment of accurate information regarding previous treatment of addiction and mental health illness and their effectiveness. This has an impact on patients' attitude, self-esteem and self-efficacy.

(4) Physical screening methods, consisting of urine toxicology for drugs and alcohol, full blood count, serum electrolyte and liver function test are carried out to establish a baseline. Hepatitis B & C and testing for HIV are discussed and arrangements are made for pre- and post-testing counselling as appropriate. A full physical examination including patients' weight and breathalyser is also undertaken. Hepatitis B vaccination is offered, if appropriate, and monitored.

Patients' desire to seek help and their motivation to change and maintain the change must be assessed as early as possible. This will require enquiries regarding patients' degree of awareness of their substance misuse/mental health problems and the connection between the two as well as the consequences of both. In addition the team should enquire whether the patient's desire to seek help is due to external or internal pressure (external such as loss of job, break up of marriage or internal such as unhappiness, anxiety, depression, lack of self-worth).

Social/family/occupation/housing and legal status should be clearly obtained. Significant others need to be involved in assessment wherever possible, in order to corroborate histories, obtain families' perspective of patient problems and assess the degree of codependency, to assist the team with risk assessment and to establish family psychopathology.

Full diagnosis (medical, psychiatric and psychodynamic formulation) is established using ICD 10 criteria and/or DSM-IV.

The patient's needs are established, and a care plan is set to address these needs. The team decides which management strategy is suitable for the patient, i.e. will they be accepted for the programme (inpatient or outpatient), will they be offered partial or alternative services (from Greenbank or away) or due to factors such as poor stability, etc., be referred back to CMHT. If the patient is admitted to their programme, a key worker is identified. Patients are required to read, agree and sign their care plan. Patients will be made aware of the unit's rules and patients' rights and responsibilities are discussed and agreed. Boundaries are fairly and firmly implemented. This tends to help the patients feel respected, safe and secure. Patients will need reassurance regarding confidentiality.

Detoxification

There is great emphasis for detoxification and mental health issues to be addressed in parallel rather than in isolation. It is the team's experience that patients with dual diagnosis require an inpatient detoxification as the most appropriate type of intervention for the following reasons:

(1) Inpatient treatment provides a drug and alcohol free setting with clear and constant boundaries that counter impulsivity and characteristic chaotic behaviour. Removal from a social environment where cues for alcohol and drug abuse are most powerful, or from a family environment where high expressed emotions may be present, which will contribute to the maintenance of addiction and mental illness.

(2) Relief and protection for families and community who may be at risk, in addition to providing a safe environment for the patient.

(3) Physical withdrawal is safely, effectively and rapidly accomplished with minimum distress to the patient who might otherwise have difficulty in complying with the detoxification regime in the community.

(4) Patients with physical and psychiatric health problems can be managed efficiently and effectively. This will reduce the risk of admission to accident and emergency or psychiatric hospitals.

(5) It creates scope for education and has been shown to contribute to good outcome (such as proceeding to more intensive treatment or remaining engaged in therapy).

(6) It provides an opportunity for the patient to focus on engaging in treatment, to develop an understanding of their problem; specifically the relationship between mental illness and addiction, and the need for detoxification and abstinence to clarify the cause and effect which in turn leads to effective management. It also allows patients to explore emotional issues and vulnerabilities, which in turn helps them focus and enhances their motivation to change.

(7) It provides opportunity for the degree of dependence as well as severity and intensity of mental health problems to be assessed in parallel and managed effectively.

196

Inpatient treatment/day programme

The next stage comprises a 6–8 week programme where a range of psychological treatment is provided through individual and group therapy. The treatment is eclectic in that it draws on elements of several different models to achieve abstinence as a main goal for therapy. These psychological treatments are part of the whole package of care and are an integral component of mental health care. The Treatment Programme consists of:

Daily group therapy (psychodynamic and cognitive behavioural)

The psychodynamic groups help patients to examine their relationships and issues underlying their symptoms and difficulties in order to achieve resolution. Cognitive behavioural groups aim to change unhelpful beliefs and attitudes, to unlearn old destructive behaviours and establish new healthy behaviour. Groups are modified specifically to meet the needs of addicts. For example, regular urine testing, breathalysing, regular attendance and group leadership (see below) are mandatory. These requirements encourage patients to take responsibility for their actions and have positive feedback from the team and other members. They also help establish boundaries and create a safe environment for patients and staff.

Group leadership tests the ability of the patient to plan and structure time effectively, to take responsibility for others, and to acknowledge the value of order in preventing disorder. Patients are required to act as group leader for a period of one week. Patients are also required to present their life story to the group. This provides an opportunity for reflection and correction and for patients to learn from shared experiences.

Key workers

Daily care planning sessions are held daily with the patient's key worker. These consist of clarifying patients' needs and ensuring that they are met. The key worker also provides individual counselling which may be solution focused, psychodynamic, problem based, motivational, or focused on relapse prevention. In addition, marital, couple and family therapy in liaison with a social worker is provided when necessary. The key worker also has the responsibility for liaison with outside bodies such as probation officers/employers on behalf of the patient.

Focus work

Additional individual sessions are provided in the form of focus sessions. These are arranged in response to specific needs, e.g. childhood sexual abuse, post traumatic stress disorder (PTSD), depressive and anxiety symptoms, etc., that are seen to contribute to the patient's difficulties. These sessions establish an emotionally and psychologically safe environment with clear boundaries where the patient is helped to establish what he/she is hoping for from treatment. It is seen as anchoring the work into the overall therapeutic response that Greenbank offers.

Relapse prevention groups

These operate on a cognitive psychotherapy model incorporating exposure to high risk situations, use of coping response, self-efficacy, outcome expectancies and abstinence violation effects.

AA-orientation/facilitation meetings

There is a weekly meeting led by an active AA (Alcoholics Anonymous) member aimed at introducing clients to the philosophy and practice of AA to allow scope for postdischarge relapse prevention.

Art and drama therapy

Weekly sessions are run by qualified art and drama therapists on a group and individual therapy basis. The therapy provides another platform for patients to explore and express feelings and issues which they have difficulty verbalising.

Partners and relatives group

These are run on a weekly basis aimed at supporting family members and explore other issues which might be relevant to ongoing treatment such as family behaviour which might help to maintain patients' addiction and/or mental illness (sick role).

Specific psychiatric treatment

Whenever indicated, weekly mental state assessment is carried out and medication reviewed. Should the patient's mental health deteriorate suddenly, arrangements are made to transfer them to CMHT for a period of further stabilisation. They are able to return to continue with the programme if possible.

Dietics and physiotherapy

Whenever indicated, appropriate arrangements for advice from a dietician and physiotherapy are made through internal referral.

Entertainment therapy

A $1\frac{1}{2}$ hour group is held 4 times a year, which combines having fun with ex-

198

posing oneself to high levels of adrenaline: both excitement and fear. The session allows people to challenge negative and automatic thoughts such as the belief that no fun can be had without alcohol. Individuals or small groups present jokes, songs or other party pieces, and staff take part wherever possible to role model coping strategies. The entertainment part of the group is followed by a short debrief session for clients to reflect on their experience and ask for help where necessary.

Programme review

A multidisciplinary care plan review takes place weekly where patients' progress is reviewed, new needs are addressed, goals redefined and discharge planned.

Day patient programme

This is a 6-week programme which enables the patients to live at home and attend Greenbank for therapeutic intervention. This programme is offered to patients with a level of support from either spouse or carer in the community and the patient should be able to demonstrate ability to sustain abstinence. It is particularly suitable for men and women with children and other domestic commitments. The option is made available on assessment and is consistent with our community care programme.

After-care

Follow-up facilities

On completion of the residential day programme, all patients are offered a minimum of two weeks follow-up programme, which consists of attending Greenbank from 9 am to 5 pm to consolidate attained objectives and set new ones.

Open meetings

This service is available as part of an abstinence/maintenance programme and is open to all ex-members who choose to participate as part of their individual strategy.

Drop-in facilities

These are counselling sessions to enable patients to deal with crisis and are offered to clients on an individual need basis. The patients are offered up to 72 hours' guesting facilities if they feel vulnerable and at risk due to his/her perception of crisis.

Reunion party/networking meeting

This takes place four times a year where ex-members meet to enjoy an informal gathering. It functions as a support social system and provides role modelling for patients in the early stages of their recovery.

Crisis intervention: volunteers/flying squad

This service is available to ex-members and carers as a relapse prevention as well as relapse management strategy. The 24 hour telephone advisory and counselling service is available to patients and carers in emotional crisis for support as well as an opportunity to select the most appropriate options including an early appointment with the team, respite care, or a visit by the flying squad members.

The service consists of former clients along with their Assertive Outreach Workers (who operate on a 9–5 basis) responding to relatives' and ex-patients' calls for assistance 24 h a day. Members of the 'flying squad' are required to have been in the abstinence stage for a minimum of one year and to have skills and strength to assist others in crisis. The volunteers receive supervision and support from a senior member of the team.

Patients are transferred to appropriate accommodation as recommended by the multidisciplinary team, whether to their own families or to alternative supportive accommodation such as dry houses. Greenbank has established good links with the Surrey Community Development Trust and other charity organisations, who provide a number of dry houses in the area. There is a two-week compulsory attendance at Greenbank following transfer to follow-up. After this, a graded disengagement from therapy takes place over a period of time depending on patients' individual needs (patients are encouraged to take an active role in this decision). As research has shown, patients do better when they remain in therapy. For this reason, patients are offered one group session per week indefinitely on relapse prevention. Attendance is voluntary. There are two additional 'open' groups per week which patients can attend, as well as drop-in and nonadmission short stay (guesting) to be used by patients in times of crisis. There is also a monthly networking evening where ex-patients are invited to the unit to provide role models for and give support to present members of the programme. Patients are encouraged to attend AA/NA meetings. Those with complex needs will receive community treatment from CMHT and CDAT teams as appropriate. Some patients will require additional long-term therapy such as counselling, psychotherapy, family therapy. These are arranged with the appropriate agency prior to discharge.

Further reading

Andrews, G., Slade, T. & Peters, L. (1999) Classification in Psychiatry. *ICD-10 Versus DSM-IV, British Journal of Psychiatry* **174**, 3–5.

Anon (1999) Addiction: mission, modes of working, and maximising the partnerships, Editorial. *Addiction* **94** (1), 5–11.

APA (1994) *Diagnostic and Statistical Manual of Mental Disorders*, 4th edn. American Psychiatric Association, Washington DC.

Bachmann, K., Moggi, F., Hirsbrunner, H., Donati, R. & Brodbeck, J. (1997) An integrated treatment program for dually diagnosed patients. *Psychiatric Services* **48** (3), 314–316.

Beck, A.T., Wright, F.D., Newman, C.F. & Liese, B.J. (1993) *Cognitive Therapy of Substance Abuse*. Guilford Press, New York.

Carey, K.B. (1989) Emerging treatment guidelines for mentally ill chemical abusers. *Hospital and Community Psychiatry* **40** (4), 341–349.

Clarke, R.E. (1996) Family support for persons with dual disorders. *New Directions for Mental Health Services* **70**, 65–78.

Cottler, L.B., Compton, W.M., Mager, D., Spitznagel, E.L. & Janca, A. (1992) Post-traumatic stress disorder among substance users from the general population. *American Journal of Psychiatry* **149** (5), 664–670.

Daley, D. (1986) *Relapse Prevention Workbook for Alcoholic Drug Dependent Persons*. Learning Publications Inc., Holmes Beach, FL.

Daley, D., Moss, H. & Campbell, F. (1987) *Dual Disorders — counselling clients with chemical dependency and mental illness*. Hazelden Foundation, Minneapolis.

Drake, R., Haas, J., Teague, G.B., Noordsy, D. & Clark, R.E. (1993) Treatment of substance abuse in severely mentally ill patients. *Journal of Nervous and Mental Diseases* **181** (10), 69–79.

Drake, R., Mueser, K.T., Clarke, R. & Wallach, M.A. (1996) The course, treatment and outcome of substance disorder in persons with severe mental illness. *American Journal of Orthopsychiatry* **66** (1), 42–51.

Duckert, F., Amundsen, A. & Johnsen, J. (1992) What happens to drinking after therapeutic intervention? *British Journal of Addiction* **87**, 1457–1467.

EATA (1997) *Treatment and Care: A New Programme for Drug and Alcohol Dependency*. European Association for the Treatment of Addiction UK, London.

El-Guebaly, N. (1900) Substance abuse and mental disorders: the dual diagnosis concept. *Canadian Journal of Psychiatry* **35**, 261–267.

El-Mallakh, P. (1998) Treatment models for clients with co-occurring addictive and mental disorders. *Archives of Psychiatric Nursing* **12** (2), 71–80.

Evans, K. & Sullivan, J.M. (1995) *Treating Addicted Survivors of Trauma*. Guilford Press, New York.

Flores, P.J. & Mahon, L. (1995) The treatment of addiction in group psychotherapy *International Journal of Group Psychotherapy* **43** (2), 43–52.

Gafoor, M. & Rassool, G. Hussein (1998) The co-existence of psychiatric disorders and substance misuse: working with dual diagnosis patients. *Journal of Advanced Nursing* **27**, 497–502.

Galanter, M., Egelko, S., Edwards, H. & Vergaray, M. (1994) A treatment system for combined psychiatric and addictive illness. *Addiction* **89**, 1227–1235, October.

Ghodse, H. (1995) *Drugs and Addictive Behaviour: a guide to treatment*, 2nd edn. Blackwell Science, Oxford.

Henningfield, J.E. & Singleton, E.G. (1994) Managing drug dependence: psychotherapy or pharmacotherapy? *CNS Drugs* **1** (5), 317–322.

Jerrell, J. & Ridgely, S. (1995a) Comparative effectiveness of three approaches to serving people with severe mental illness and substance misuse disorder. *Journal of Nervous and Mental Disease* **183**, 566–576.

Jerrell, J. & Ridgely, M. (1995b) Evaluation changes in symptoms and functioning of dually diagnosed clients in specialised treatment. *Psychiatric Services* **46** (3), 233–237.

Johnson, S. (1997) Dual diagnosis of severe mental illness and substance misuse: a case for specialist services? *British Journal of Psychiatry* **171**, 205–208.

Kaufman, E. (1997) Family therapy: a treatment approach with substance abusers. In: J.H. Lowinson, P. Ruiz, R.B. Millman & J.G. Lan (eds) *Substance Abuse: a Comprehensive Textbook*, 2nd edn. Williams & Wilkins, Baltimore.

Khantzian, E.J. (1990) Self-regulation and self-medication factors in alcoholism and addictions; similarities and differences. In: M. Galanter (ed.) *Recent Developments in Alcoholism*, Vol. 8. Plenum Press, New York, pp. 255–269.

Khantzian, E.J., Halliday, K.S., Golden, S. & McAuliffe, W.E. (1992) Modified group therapy for substance abusers, a psychodynamic approach to relapse prevention. *American Journal on Addictions*. Winter.

McHugo, G., Drake, R., Burton, H. & Ackerson, T. (1995) A scale for assessing the stage of substance abuse treatment in persons with severe mental illness. *Journal of Nervous and Mental Disease* **183** (12), 762–767.

Mee-Lee, D. & Shulman, G.D. (1999) Towards Clinically Effective and Cost Efficient, Outcomes-Driven Treatment. NCADD—Committee on Treatment Benefits, www.ncadd.org.

Miller, N. (1994) Psychiatric comorbidity: occurrence and treatment. *Alcohol Health Research World* **18** (4), 261–263.

Miller, W.R. & Rollnick, S. (1991) Motivational interviewing. *Preparing People to Change Addictive Behaviour*. Guilford Press, New York.

Minkoff, K. (1989) An integrated treatment model for dual diagnosis. *Hospital and Community Psychiatry* **40**, 1031–1036.

Moos, R. & Moos, B. (1995) Stay in residential facilities and mental health care as predictors of readmission for patients with substance use disorders. *Psychiatric Services* **46** (1), 66–72.

Najavits, L.M. & Weiss, R.D. (1994) The role of psychotherapy in the treatment of substance-use disorders. *Harvard Review of Psychiatry* July/August.

NHS Executive (1995) *Reviewing Shared Care Arrangements for Drug Users*, Circular no. **95**, 114. Department of Health, London.

N.I.D.A. (National Institute on Drug Abuse) (1991) Third Biennial Report to Congress: Drug Abuse and Drug Abuse Research. Cited by M. Gafoor & G.H. Rassool (1998) The co-existence of psychiatric disorders and substance misuse: working with dual diagnosis patients. *Journal of Advanced Nursing* **27** (3), 497–502.

Pechter, B.M. & Miller, N.S. (1997) Psychopharmacotherapy for addictive and co-morbid disorders: current studies. *Journal of Addictive Diseases* **16** (4), 23–40.

Peele, S. (2000) *Denial—of Reality and of Freedom*. www.peele.net.

Priestley, J.S., Rassool, G. Hussein, Saffer, D. & Ghodse, H.A. (1998) Psychodynamic psychotherapy and counselling: what contribution can it make to the treatment of addiction? *Journal of Substance Misuse* **3**, 234–239.

Prochaska, J.O., DiClimente, C.C. & Norcross, C. (1992) In search of how people change: applications to addictive behavior. *American Psychologist* **47**, 1102–1114.

Rassool, G.H. (1993) Nursing and substance misuse: responding to the challenge. *Journal of Advanced Nursing* **18**, 1401–1407.

Read, A. (1991) Addiction. In: J. Holmes (ed.) *Textbook of Psychotherapy in Psychiatric Practice*. Churchill Livingstone, Edinburgh.

Ries, R., Mullen, M. & Cox, G. (1994) Symptom severity and utilisation of treatment resources among dually diagnosed inpatients. *Hospital and Community Psychiatry* **45** (6), 562–567.

Riordan, R.J. (1992) The use of mirror image therapy in substance abuse groups. *Journal of Counseling & Development* **71**, September/October.

Rorstad, P. & Checinski, K. (1996) *Dual Diagnosis: Facing the Challenge*. Wynne Howard Publishing, Kenley.

Rosenheck, R., Massari, L., Astrachan, B. & Suchinsky, R. (1990) Mentally ill chemical abusers discharged from VA inpatient treatment. *Psychiatric Quarterly* **61**, 237–249.

Rounsaville, B.J. & Carroll, K.M. (1994) Individual psychotherapy for drug abusers. In: J.H. Lowinson, P. Ruiz, R.B. Millman & J.G. Lan (eds) *Substance Abuse: a Comprehensive Textbook*, 2nd edn. Williams & Wilkins, Baltimore.

Rubinstein, L., Campbell, F. & Daley, D. (1990) Four perspectives on dual diagnosis: an overview of treatment issues. *Journal of Chemical Dependency Treatment* **3** (2), 97–118.

Stark, M.J. (1992) Dropping out of substance abuse treatment: a clinically oriented review. *Clinical Psychology Review* **12**, 93–116.

Surrey Social Services Department (1998) *Development of a Programme of Care for People with a Dual Diagnosis of Mental Illness and Substance Misuse.* A report by Rorstad Associates, London.

Teague, G., Drake, R. & Ackerson, T. (1995) Evaluating use of continuous treatment teams for persons with mental illness and substance abuse. *Psychiatric Services* **46** (7), 689–695.

Tolsma, R.J., Driol, M.E. & Hiland, T.A. (1992) Psychotherapy and addiction: a survey of journals. *International Journal of the Addictions* **27** (11), 1249–1266.

Tomasson, K. & Vaglum, P. (1995) A nationwide representative sample of treatment-seeking alcoholics: a study of psychiatric comorbidity. *Acta Psychiatrica Scandinavia* **92**, 378–385.

White, R.K. & Wright, D.G., eds (1999) Addiction Intervention: Strategies to Motivate Treatment-Seeking Behavior. www.therapeuticresources.com.

Wilson, J. (1998) Dual diagnosis: addiction and CSA, The Scottish Drugs Training Project has found compelling reasons for addiction services to re-evaluate their practices. *ACW Magazine* May/June.

Young, N.K. & Grella, C.E. (1998) Mental health and substance abuse treatment services for dually diagnosed clients; results of a state-wide survey of county administrators. *Journal of Behavioural Health Services and Research* **25** (1), 83–92.

Zweben, J.E. (1993a) Dual diagnosis—key issues for the 1990s (reprinted from *Psychology of Addictive Behaviors*). *International Journal of Psychosocial Rehabilitation* **7** (3), 168–172. www.psychosocial.com.

Zweben, J.E. (1993b) Recovery oriented psychotherapy: a model for addiction treatment. *Psychotherapy* **30**.

16: Dual or Separate Services?

James Edeh

Introduction

The expanding literature on dual diagnosis is matched equally by the lack of agreement on a model of service that has universal acceptance. The term 'dual disorder' or *dual diagnosis* is now used interchangeably with *comorbidity* of psychiatric and substance use disorders. Feinstein (1970) used the term 'comorbidity' to imply the co-occurrence of distinct clinical entities. Minkoff (1989) in agreement with most researchers and clinicians, restricted dual diagnosis only to patients who have substance abuse or dependence and a primary psychotic illness, such as schizophrenia or a major effective disorder (bipolar or unipolar) as defined in DSM-III-R Axis I disorders (APA 1987). Considerable controversy exists about the inclusion of Axis II disorders and some doubts also cloud Axis I disorders (Verheul *et al.* 2000). A substance-related artifact hypothesis has evolved and begs the question whether recovery from substance use disorders co-occur with recovery from mood/anxiety or personality disorders at rates exceeding those predicted by chance. Ghodse (1995) remarked that personality disorders are associated with a higher severity of substance use, and do not readily yield to symptom-specific interventions. In a concise but stimulating editorial, Hall and Farrell (1997) summed up the main epidemiological findings derived largely from Regier *et al.* (1990); the rates of co-occurrence of psychiatric and substance use disorders varying between 20% and 50% depending on the survey population.

This chapter reviews the argument for and against dual diagnosis service models, based on experiences in the USA, and offers an alternative approach compatible with the mental health system in the UK.

Scale of service delivery problems

Dual diagnosis patients are a heterogeneous population; the demand they make on services poses huge challenges to the health care delivery system. Exacerbation of psychotic symptoms by alcohol and/or illicit drugs is generally recognised and probably mediated through the dopamine system, a vulnerability that is particularly associated with psycho-stimulant drug use. Superimposed on this biochemical vulnerability is medication non-compliance, both factors acting together to increase relapse rates, frequent hospitalisation, chronicity and poor clinical outcomes, among dual diagnosis patients compared with those who do not have a comorbid diagnosis. It seems far-fetched however, to conclude that the diagnostic complexity associated with the co-occurrence of psychiatric and substance use disorders, without environmental and social factors, explains all the service delivery problems that have been documented. Studies of de-institutionalisation and discharge of chronic mentally ill patients to the community (Leff & Vaughan 1972; Johnstone *et al.* 1984) suggest that the service delivery problems associated with dual diagnosis today were those that had been predicted would happen with the failure of care in the community.

The discharge of individuals with chronic mental illness to the community without adequate supportive environment is compounded by their failure to engage in follow-up care, non-compliance with medication, ethnic and socio-economic disadvantage, which in association with substance use, lead to a marked predilection for aggressive and violent behaviour, and criminality; the cause–effect relationship is poorly understood.

Models of dual diagnosis services

Services have evolved over the past decade in response to the multiple needs of dual diagnosis patients, without the results of outcome studies (Ries 1992). Models of intervention are based on whether the services are identified as *separate*, that is provided by separate treatment teams, or *dual*, where one specialised team responds to both the psychiatric and substance related needs of patients.

Separate services imply the provision of care by separate teams in separate treatment facilities and management structures. There are two recognised models:

(1) The *serial* or sequential model in which one treatment follows the other but are not offered simultaneously.

(2) The *parallel* model, in which the treatments are given concurrently by the participating clinical teams.

In both models, expertise is not shared across teams. Both models have difficulties engaging patients in treatment and reducing non-compliance, which in turn is associated with poor service coordination, and fragmentation of the care delivery process. The lack of service coordination results in unmet needs as the patient is bounced between clinical teams, and eventually falls between service cracks, and drops out of treatment altogether.

A dual or *integrated* service is designed to offer a comprehensive range of interventions which include pharmacological, psycho-educational, behavioural, case management and self-help approaches. The argument in favour of the integrated model is built on the premise that it offers continuity of care, and promotes a blending of clinical expertise and enhancement of clinical skills among health care professionals in the team. Despite the expressed optimism about the integrated model, the high concentration of *difficult to treat* patients and concentration of expertise in one team are likely to isolate staff from other local services with consequences of sagging morale, disillusionment and burn-out. There are also issues related to the costs of integrating specialised services and the level of staffing that would be required if a key worker or case manager is assigned only a small caseload of *difficult to treat* patients; many district teams, in the face of an ever-increasing demand for services and static or dwindling resources, do not have this leverage.

Separate services

The limitations of separate services reside in the failure to significantly engage patients in treatment, promote retention and prevent relapse. These problems are compounded by differing treatment philosophies across clinical teams and therapeutic objectives which fail to recognise graded goals and a continuum of outcomes for substance use, from harm reduction to total abstinence. Both the serial (sequential) and parallel (concurrent) models often result in fragmented, contradictory and inadequate care (Drake *et al.* 1993): both models of services maximise the potential for ineffective delivery of care, non-compliance and treatment drop-out.

The integrated model

What does it offer?

Conceptual problems arise because there is no consistent package of interventions to which the term *integrated* can be ascribed. From the care delivery perspective, excluding service funding and management structures, the dominant issues are about:
- integrated teams
- integrated service components and
- integrated treatment principles and philosophies.

Integrated teams

An argument which lends support to an integrated service model is the suggested effectiveness of multidisciplinary teams (referred to as continuous treatment teams), which take responsibility for small caseloads of *difficult to treat* patients, and offer active intervention, such as outreach in the community, engagement in treatment, intensive supervision and close monitoring, with some impact on treatment compliance and rehabilitation. Drake *et al.* (1990) developed this approach successfully to engage and retain patients with dual diagnosis in long-term treatment in New Hampshire, by combining intensive case management with assertive outreach.

Though Drake *et al.* (1993) argued that the costs involved in integrating substance abuse treatment into community mental health programmes, either through case managers or continuous treatment teams, are minimal, Godley *et al.* (2000) have highlighted some of the difficulties involved in intensive case management of dually diagnosed individuals; the authors observed variations in the job descriptions of case managers, because they worked for different agencies, and in the event of a leave of absence, a case manager could not easily stand in for another; that at times their interface with clients served different purposes and there were no standard procedures for working with families and significant others.

Despite the theoretical merits of intensive case management and assertive outreach, there are organisational problems in the service delivery process and deriving maximum benefits therapeutically for patients. The UK 700 case management trial of the cost-effectiveness of intensive vs. standard case management for severe psychotic illness (UK 700 Group 2000) concluded that reduced caseloads have no clear beneficial effect on costs, clinical outcomes or indeed cost-effectiveness; the results of this study of 708 patients with psychosis, randomly allocated to standard (caseloads 30–35) or intensive (caseloads 10–15) did not lend support to the intensive case management approach.

Integrated service components

Service components of the integrated model show marked variations, with the notable exception of the 12-step self-help programme, which appears a consistent therapeutic adjunct, irrespective of the setting (see Table 16.1).

The trend through the 1990s was a decline in optimism about the integrated service model. Lehman *et al.* (1993) compared an experimental group ($n=29$) and control group ($n=25$) of patients with dual diagnosis, randomly assigned to the community mental health centre (CMHC) and rehabilitation services, with or without on-site self-help group and intensive case management; the results were disappointing at one year follow-up: there was a notable lack of improvement on most outcome measures. Bartels and Drake (1996) carried out a process evaluation and six-month outcome study of a residential dual diagnosis treatment programme based on an integrated model; improvement at follow-up was unrelated to successful programme completion.

Ridgely and Jerrell (1996) carried out a qualitative study of three service components often included in the integrated model—intensive case management (ICM), behavioural skills training (BST) and a 12-step Alcoholics Anonymous (AA)/Narcotics Anonymous (NA) social recovery approach; the authors observed that the AA groups varied across participating agencies, in the supportive experience offered to clients; there was also a wide variation in the skills level and enthusiasm of CMHC staff for the BST intervention and higher caseloads interfered with case managers' ability to provide intensive service to their clients. In summary, Ridgely and Jerrell (1996) observed that the model *implementation* differed from the programme *design*.

Integrated treatment principles and philosophies

Minkoff (1989) argued that an integrated treatment philosophy would remove the conflict which arises when addiction and mental health treatment programmes try to collaborate. Table 16.2 provides an outline of principles and philosophies which have been identified for effective treatment of addictive disorders (Waltman 1995) and dual diagnosis (Drake *et al.* 1993). The principles and philosophies themselves have some sound rational basis, but their application in practice in the management of comorbid disorders face several pitfalls.

An obvious questions is—do treatment philosophies need to be integrated to be responsive to patients' needs or is it possible to accommodate differing treatment philosophies in a model that is not integrated but responds better to the needs of patients? Carey (1996) addressed this question admirably in her proposed collaborative approach which allows for a flexibility in treatment goals, and accommodates a harm minimisation rather than an abstinence-only, zero-tolerance philosophy. The sets of treatment principles and philosophies of both Waltman (1995) and Drake *et al.* (1993) actually

Table 16.1 Integrated service components

Authors	Treatment settings	Service components	Outcome evaluation
Kofoed *et al.* (1986)	Outpatients; Portland VA Medical Centre, USA	90 minute weekly group; prescribed medication AA/NA meetings	High drop-out rate: only 33% retention at 3 months follow-up
Hellerstein and Meehan (1987)	Outpatients; Beth Israel Medical Centre Prescribed medication	Once-a-week group therapy open ended; AA/NA meetings	Marked decrease in days of hospitalisation at one-year follow-up
Greenfield *et al.* (1995)	Inpatient, 180-bed unit McLean Hospital Harvard Medical School, USA	A consultation liaison service supportive non-confrontational group; follow-up at discharge	Evaluation of outcome: none
Franco *et al.* (1995)	Inpatient setting in New York, USA approach	Token economy programme and a 12-step self-help discharge	Decrease in violence and self-injury but follow-up after proved problematic
Lehman *et al.* (1993)	CMHC and rehabilitation Baltimore, Maryland, USA	Demonstration project with experimental group (n=29) and control (n=25) assigned to CMHC and rehab services with/without on-site self-help group and intensive case management	Follow-up at one year was disappointing; notable lack of change on most outcome measures
Bartels and Drake (1996)	Pond Place, 12-bed residential programme, New Hampshire, USA	Mental health care and addiction treatment; daily psychotherapy group; 12-step, self-help meetings	Improvement was unrelated at six months to successful programme completion

Table 16.2 Integrated treatment principles and philosophies

Addictive disorders Waltman (1995)	Dual diagnosis Drake *et al.* (1993)
1. Easy accessibility	Assertiveness
2. Treatment flexibility	Flexibility and specialisation
3. Collateral involvement	Stable living situation
4. Good therapist	Optimism
5. Motivated clients	Close monitoring
6. Matching treatment to client variables	Comprehensiveness
7. Client accountability for their sobriety	Stages of treatment
8. Focused treatment approaches	Integration
9. Follow-up	Longitudinal perspective

The order of listing does not suggest similarities or differences.

accommodate treatment flexibility and a longitudinal perspective; however, in practice within a dual or integrated approach, these are not readily achievable.

Minkoff (1989) also indicated that the legal system may be necessary for a patient's engagement in treatment to succeed. Osher and Kofoed (1989) gave supportive evidence that coercive treatment has been associated with improved programme retention among dual diagnosis patients. Under the Mental Health Act, 1983 in the UK, it would be inappropriate to enforce engagement or compliance on grounds of substance abuse or dependence, except only in circumstances of altered mental state where insight or capacity for rational decision making is impaired and compulsory detention and/or treatment is indicated for the protection of the individual or the public (Bluglass & Rawnsley 1983). An integrated service model for the care of dual diagnosis patients in the UK would have legal shortcomings; the indication of a section of the Mental Health Act, 1983, whether for reasons of substance use disorder or exacerbation of a psychotic state would become inextricably intertwined.

Concerns that some agencies would have about the biological theory of addiction and a biological approach to treatment and care are discussed under the subheading *integrating psychotherapy and pharmacotherapy.*

Miscellaneous and related issues

A number of issues deserve specific mention; these are:
integrating psychotherapy and pharmacotherapy
nicotine dependence in the context of dual diagnosis
ethnic differences in service utilisation.

Integrating psychotherapy and pharmacotherapy

There are undoubtedly therapeutic benefits in combining pharmacological and non-pharmacological interventions, but providing these treatments within an integrated service model for dual disorders poses some problems. A 12-step self-help programme, cognitive-behavioural and motivational approaches are routinely available within the addiction services with minor modifications and variations. Pharmacologically assisted detoxification in alcohol dependence using diazepam or chlormethiazole reducing regimes, or for opiate withdrawal using methadone, clonidine, naltrexone or buprenorphine, or alleviation of withdrawal symptoms in smoking cessation with nicotine replacement therapy (NRT) are well established. The use of neuroleptic and/or antidepressant medication in co-occurring disorders is certain to lengthen the list of prescribed medication with resulting polypharmacy and iatrogenic consequences. Very little is known about polypharmacy as a possible explanation for medication non-compliance or episodes of self-poisoning among dual diagnosis patients. Rational prescribing though acknowledged and talked about is not readily achievable; there are major risks from misuse of prescribed drugs. Ghodse *et al.* (1985) reported in the Home Office study of deaths of drug addicts in the United Kingdom, from 1967 to 1981, that in most deaths of non-therapeutic addicts in which a drug was implicated, 74% were due to medically prescribed drugs.

In the UK, most non-statutory treatment agencies are opposed to the biological theory of the addictions and rely largely on psychosocial interventions. The results of Project MATCH (Project MATCH Research Group 1997) should come as good news to alcohol abuse treatment agencies which favour a predominantly non-pharmacological approach. Project MATCH compared a 12-step facilitation therapy (TSF), a 12-session cognitive-behaviour therapy (CBT) and a motivational enhancement therapy (MET); patients in all three treatment groups showed improvement in their reduced consumption of alcohol, abstinence rates and psychosocial functioning. Therefore integrating pharmacotherapy with psychotherapy should apply selectively for resolution of acute psychotic symptoms, or use of depot preparations of psychotropic medication for chronicity, even where substitution therapy on a maintenance basis for substance use disorders is indicated.

Psychotherapy when combined sensibly with pharmacotherapy should avoid polypharmacy. Restricted prescribing would reduce untoward drug reactions, toxicity and self-poisoning episodes, and abuse of medication which have a dependence potential.

Nicotine dependence in the context of dual diagnosis

Nicotine dependence is common among psychiatric patients (Ziedonis *et al.* 1994). There is a relationship between cigarette smoking and affective disorder, particularly depression. It is also known that smoking cigarettes may trigger cravings for other substances, such as cocaine and alcohol. Researchers and service providers should establish objectives and strategies for treating nicotine dependence among patients with major mental disorders.

Ethnic differences in service utilisation

The prevalence of dual diagnosis among ethnic minority groups has attracted attention. Jerrell and Wilson (1997) examined psychosocial functioning, psychiatric disorder and substance use among whites and three ethnic groups comprising African-Americans, Asian-Americans and Hispanics; the non-white ethnic groups had lower psychosocial functioning scores and received less supportive treatment services.

In a multicultural environment, the need for more ethnically diverse staff to deliver services and the removal of institutional barriers to service utilisation add to the long list of challenges in developing a model of service easily accessible to all social groups irrespective of demographic and socio-economic background.

Liaison or collaborative service model?

Quite apart from the lack of evidence for effectiveness of the integrated model, such an approach to the care of dual diagnosis patients in the UK would result in a disruption to the catchment area responsibilities of community mental health teams (CMHTs), community drug teams (CDTs), and community alcohol teams (CATs). Their operational policies and working arrangements, budgetary structures and a dilution of practices, protocols and procedures developed within individual teams over many years. The constitution of addiction services also varies enormously across districts, from a walk-in advice and counselling service, with or without a prescribing component provided by general practitioners, to a specialised or highly specialised range of statutory or non-statutory services. The contribution from the private sector is growing but remains relatively small and largely detached from mainstream mental health and addiction treatment services. Integrated teams, budgets, service components and their management and treatment philosophies would pose enormous problems.

There is agreement that the serial model fosters therapeutic nihilism, and therefore has no place in the management of dual diagnosis patients. The parallel model suffers from a lack of service coordination, shared expertise among professionals, a joint approach to the delivery of care, joint monitoring, interagency collaboration and a programme of multi-professional training which provides opportunities for clinicians to learn new skills and modify their attitudes. A liaison and collaborative service model has the potential to address all these issues.

Ridgely *et al.* (1998) reported some evidence in support of inter-agency collaboration, *collaboratives* or communities of providers working together to offer coordinated mental health and substance abuse treatment and support. Evaluation at one-year and two years of one such collaborative in the state of Maine, USA, showed an increase in interagency referrals, joint assessment of patients, jointly sponsored multi-professional training and joint funding for service provision. One advantage of a liaison and collaborative model is that it fosters service coordination without smothering treatment philosophies or imposing ideologies which a treatment agency involved in the *partnership* or *collaborative* finds difficult to embrace. Carey (1996) described a collaborative, motivational approach which accommodates a harm minimisation philosophy for reducing substance use and risk behaviours without a rigid adherence to an abstinence-only, zero-tolerance goal. Rosenheck *et al.* (1998) added a touch of realism to the debate on the costs of highly specialised treatment programmes, which do not offer continuity and consistency of care because of resource limitations and are not easily accessible to patients. A huge argument in support of a liaison and collaborative model is that it could be designed to fit the level of resources available within individual districts and the prevailing local circumstances, and it could also be designed to respond flexibly to change over time, such that the service keeps pace with demand and trend.

The liaison and collaborative service model requires a health district to set up a Dual Diagnosis Management Team comprising care professionals elected from each of the CMHTs operating within the district and representatives from the addiction services, with the remit to review dual diagnosis cases known to district teams fortnightly or once monthly, in a case conference setting , and with feedback to individual teams on recommended action plans, specific communication to respective key workers on progress or the lack of it in the care delivery process and any proposed changes to care plans. The case conference setting also provides a forum for multi-professional and shared learning, interchange or ideas on treatment philosophies and the erosion of institutional barriers.

There may be variations in the terms of reference and composition of dual diagnosis management teams across health districts, to include or co-opt key staff, or encourage participation from the social services, housing department, probation service and the advocacy service. Clearly a database of all dual diagnosis cases in every health district kept and maintained by the dual diagnosis management team would assist monitoring, promote proactive intervention and prevent patients falling through cracks in the care delivery system.

In the UK, admission of dual diagnosis patients to general psychiatric wards has been a practice over 30 years, even at a time when the planned closure of large mental hospitals was beginning to gather momentum. The idea of a dual diagnosis specific inpatient programme (Franco *et al.* 1995) smacks of *double stigmatisation* and is not helpful in promoting patients' self-image and self-confidence. Inpatient care for individuals with dual diagnosis in a psychiatric ward was routine practice at Tooting Bec Hospital in South London, England before it closed. Since the early 1980s, patients with dual diagnosis have been and continue to be admitted to John Meyer Ward and Bluebell Ward, which are both acute psychiatric wards at Springfield University Hospital in Tooting, London. Since 1988, patients with dual diagnosis have been routinely admitted to Rose Ward at Horsham Hospital and the Villa Ward at the Princess Royal Hospital, Haywards Heath; both of which are open psychiatric wards in Sussex, south-east England. These are only a few examples of good practice, based on well developed protocols and operational procedures. Therefore, the challenge facing health care professionals is not the provision of hospitalisation when required, but the effectiveness of follow-up at discharge and after-care programmes. Reed (1997) stressed that the use of the Care Programme Approach (CPA) (Department of Health 1990) for implementing care plans and monitoring patients' progress through reviews of the care plans cannot be over-emphasised. Assessment of risk should be an ongoing process and should be accompanied by risk management, an obligation under clinical governance (Royal College of Physicians 2000).

The success of a liaison and collaborative model will depend also on the number of settings patients are expected to attend for treatment and care. Excluding the domiciliary setting and the general practice setting, a patient should not be required to attend more than two other treatment settings in the outpatient department, day hospital or community-based location. Expecting patients to attend treatment at multiple venues often results in failure to engage, non-compliance and drop-out.

The institutional and organisational structures for health service funding, management and interagency partnerships in the UK are different from those in the USA. All the tools necessary to guarantee adequate care for dual diagnosis patients, ensure their safety and protect the public already exist within the mental health system in the UK. The challenge to health care professionals is how to employ these tools and apply them responsibly and effectively through liaison and collaboration.

Conclusion

There is agreement amongst clinicians and researchers that neither the serial (sequential) nor the parallel (concurrent) model of service offers dual diagnosis patients a realistic prospect of treatment effectiveness. The search however, for a better service model has been equally disappointing: current trends lend support to a liaison and collaborative model with the potential to blend clinical expertise across teams, harness various service components (Ridgely *et al.* 1998) and accommodate differing treatment philosophies (Carey 1996). Despite the therapeutic optimism of the late 1980s about an integrated service model, Ridgely and Jerrell (1996) observed that studies designed to evaluate such integrated programmes have not demonstrated proven effectiveness and that most lacked relevant details. The findings of their qualitative study, summed up in *the gap between expectation and performance,* exposed a *drift* between the design of treatment programmes and *fidelity* in implementation.

References

American Psychiatric Association (1987) *Diagnostic and Statistical Manual of Mental Disorders*, 3rd edn revised. American Psychiatric Association, Washington DC.

Bartels, S.J. & Drake, R.E. (1996) A pilot study of residential treatment for dual diagnoses. *Journal of Nervous and Mental Disease* **184**, 379–351.

Bluglass, R. & Rawnsley, K. (1983) *A Guide to the Mental Health Act 1983*. Churchill Livingstone, Edinburgh.

Carey, K.B. (1996) Substance use reduction in the context of outpatient psychiatric treatment: a collaborative, motivational, harm reduction approach. *Community Mental Health Journal* **32**, 291–306.

Department of Health (1990) The care programme approach for people with a mental illness referred to the specialist psychiatric service, HC (90) 23/LASSL (90) 11. Department of Health, London.

Drake, R.E., Bartels, S.J., Teague, G.B., Noordsy, D.L. & Clark, R.E. (1993) Treatment of substance abuse in severely mentally ill patients. *Journal of Nervous and Mental Disease* **181**, 606–611.

Drake, R.E., Teague, G.B. & Warren, R.S. (1990) New Hampshire dual diagnosis program for people with severe mental illness and substance use disorders. *Addiction Recovery* **10**, 35–39.

Feinstein, A.R. (1970) The pre-therapeutic classification of comorbidity in chronic disease. *Journal of Chronic Diseases* **23**, 455–468.

Franco, H., Galanter, M., Castaneda, R. & Patterson, J. (1995) Combining behavioural and self-help approaches in the inpatient management of dually diagnosed patients. *Journal of Substance Abuse Treatment* **12**, 227–232.

Ghodse, A.H., Sheehan, M., Taylor, C. & Edwards, G. (1985) Deaths of drug addicts in the United Kingdom, 1967–81. *British Medical Journal* **290**, 425–428.

Ghodse, H. (1995) Substance misuse and personality disorders: editorial review. *Current Opinion in Psychiatry* **8**, 177–179.

Godley, S.H., Finch, M., Dougan, L., McDonnell, M., McDermeit, M. & Cary, A. (2000) Case management for dually diagnosed individuals involved in the criminal justice system. *Journal of Substance Abuse Treatment* **18**, 137–148.

Greenfield, S.F., Weiss, R.D. & Tohen, M. (1995) Substance abuse and the chronically mentally ill; a description of dual diagnosis treatment services in a hospital. *Community Mental Health Journal* **31**, 265–277.

Hall, W. & Farrell, M. (1997) Comorbidity of mental disorders with substance misuse. *British Journal of Psychiatry* **171**, 4–5.

Hellerstein, D.J. & Meehan, B. (1987) Outpatient group therapy for schizophrenic substance abusers. *American Journal of Psychiatry* **144**, 1337–1339.

Jerrell, J.M. & Wilson, J.L. (1997) Ethnic differences in the treatment of dual mental and substance disorders. *Journal of Substance Abuse Treatment* **14**, 133–140.

Johnstone, C., Owens, D.G.C., Gold, A., Crow, T.J. & MacMillan, J.F. (1984) Schizophrenic patients discharged from hospital—a follow-up study. *British Journal of Psychiatry* **145**, 586–590.

Kofoed, L., Kania, J., Walsh, T. & Atkinson, R.M. (1986) Outpatient treatment of patients with substance abuse and co-existing psychiatric disorders. *American Journal of Psychiatry* **143**, 867–872.

Leff, J.P. & Vaughan, C. (1972) Psychiatric patients in contact and out of contact with services: a clinical and social assessment. In: J.K. Wing & A.M. Hailey (eds) *Evaluating a Community Psychiatric Service*. Oxford University Press, London.

Lehman, A.F., Herron, J.D., Schwartz, R.P. & Myers, C.P. (1993) Rehabilitation of adults with severe mental illness and substance use disorders. *Journal of Nervous and Mental Disease* **181**, 86–90.

Minkoff, K. (1989) An integrated treatment model for dual diagnosis of psychosis and addiction. *Hospital and Community Psychiatry* **40**, 1031–1036.

214

Osher, F.C. & Kofoed, L.L. (1989) Treatment of patients with psychiatric and psychoactive substance abuse disorders. *Hospital and Community Psychiatry* **40**, 1025–1030.

Project MATCH Research Group (1997) Matching alcoholism treatments to client heterogeneity. Project MATCH post-treatment drinking outcomes. *Journal of Studies on Alcohol* **58**, 7–29.

Reed, J. (1997) Risk assessment and clinical risk management: the lessons from recent inquiries. *British Journal of Psychiatry* **170** (Suppl. 32), 4–7.

Regier, D.A., Famer, M.E., Rae, D.S., Locke, B.Z., Keith, S.J., Judd, L.J. & Goodwin, F.K. (1990) Comorbidity of mental disorders with alcohol and other drug abuse: results from the Epidemiologic Catchment Area (ECA) study. *Journal of the American Medical Association* **264**, 2511–2518.

Ridgely, M.S. & Jerrell, J.M. (1996) Analysis of three interventions for substance abuse treatment of severely mentally ill people. *Community Mental Health Journal* **32**, 561–572.

Ridgely, M.S., Lambert, D., Goodman, A., Chichester, C. & Ralph, R. (1998) Inter-agency collaboration in services for people with co-occurring mental illness and substance use disorder. *Psychiatric Services* **49**, 236–238.

Ries, R.K. (1992) Serial, parallel and integrated models of dual-diagnosis treatment. *Journal of Health Care for the Poor and Underserved* **3**, 173–180.

Rosenheck, R., Harkness, L., Johnson, B., Sweeney, C., Buck, N., Deegan, D. & Kosten, T. (1998) Intensive community-focused treatment of Veterans with dual diagnoses. *American Journal of Psychiatry* **155**, 1429–1433.

Royal College of Physicians (2000) *Effective Clinical Risk Management in Mental Health*, Conference handbook. The Royal College of Physicians, London.

UK 700 Group (2000) Cost-effectiveness of intensive v. standard case management for severe psychotic illness. *British Journal of Psychiatry* **176**, 537–543.

Verheul, R., Kranzler, H.R., Poling, J., Tennen, H., Ball, S. & Rounsaville, B.J. (2000) Axis I and Axis II disorders in alcoholics and drug addicts: fact or artifact. *Journal of Studies on Alcohol* **61**, 101–110.

Waltman, D. (1995) Key ingredients to effective addictions treatment. *Journal of Substance Abuse Treatment* **12**, 429–439.

Ziedonis, D.M., Kosten, T.R., Glazer, W.M. & Frances, R.J. (1994) Nicotine dependence and schizophrenia. *Hospital and Community Psychiatry* **45**, 204–206.

17: Professional Education in Addiction and Mental Health Issues: A Case for Less Diagnosis and More Action?

G. Hussein Rassool

Introduction

There is an increasingly recognised problem of drug and alcohol misuse among people with mental health problems as reflected in the previous chapters. The argument for raising the profile of both substance misuse and mental health problems is challenging in the light of meeting the health targets as identified in the Health of the Nation documents (Department of Health 1992, 1993). Since substance misuse is more likely to be the norm than the exception among mentally ill patients, there is a pressing need for mental health professionals to develop their knowledge and clinical expertise in substance misuse in order to respond effectively to the needs of this group of patients. However, education and training in substance use and dual diagnosis have been largely patchy and limited; and have lagged behind the growth in service provision. Many reports have recommended that professional bodies in health and social work continue to design training in the early identification of drug and alcohol misuse and appropriate referral skills for professionals working in health, social care and criminal justice system.

That dual diagnosis education and training is an important step in the long-term strategy for improving the quality of care for those with mental health and substance use problems is beyond dispute. The goal of education and training in substance use and mental health problems must be to:

(1) provide an increased awareness and recognition of the needs of the patients;

(2) enhance the share cared and collaborative approaches between the different disciplines;

(3) improve the evidence-based intervention strategies required in dealing with such complex problems; and

(4) provide high quality care for those with dual diagnosis.

The aims of this chapter are to provide a brief review of recommendations made by the governmental agencies, advisory bodies and institutions and an overview of the current educational programme. In addition, the types of education and training and those who need training will be examined. Finally a framework for dual diagnosis courses at foundation and advanced level will be presented.

Review of recommendations: education and training

Several governmental reports have identified the importance and the need for the educational preparation of health and social care professional and allied disciplines in working with substance misusers. The reports included in this section are presented in the context of education and training of health and social care professionals. The Health of the Nation (Department of Health 1993) recommended that professional bodies in health and social work continue to promote the early identification of alcohol misuse, drug misuse and issues around sexuality and drug misuse. In *Tackling Drugs Together* (Department of Health 1994a), the document identified the importance of staff different agencies, including primary health care workers and staff in the prison health system, receiving adequate training in substance use education. The White paper *Tackling Drugs to Build a Better Britain* (Cabinet Office 1998) is the government's 10-year strategy for tackling drug misuse. The strategy has four principal aims: to help young people resist drug misuse in order to achieve their full potential in society; to protect our communities from drug-related antisocial and criminal behaviour; to enable people with drug problems to overcome them and live healthy and crime-free lives; and to stifle the availability of illegal drugs on our streets The aim of the government strategy is 'to take effective action by vigorous law enforcement, accessible treatment and a new emphasis on education and prevention'. This comprehensive initiative and approach to tackle the problem of substance misuse has a clear focus on education and prevention strategies and involves a coordinated approach both locally and nationally. (Department of Health 1992); The Advisory Council on the Misuse of Drugs (ACMD 1988; ACMD 1990, 1991; ACMD 1991) reports recommended that information on the recognition and management of drug misusers should be part of the basic training of all professionals who are likely to have contact with them. The reports further recommended that relevant training bodies take steps to ensure that appropriate arrangements for training are instituted as a matter of urgency.

The 1990 ACMD report *Problem Drug Use: A Review of Training* recommended that the appropriate professional bodies in the fields of medicine, nursing, pharmacy, psychology, social work and the criminal justice system and other related professionals should include joint training in alcohol and drugs covering appropriate attitudes, knowledge and basic management skills. The integration of substance use and misuse should be part of the core curriculum at both undergraduate and postgraduate levels. The report made further recommendation that specialist training should equip those who are directly involved in the management of drug-related problems to embrace a whole range of knowledge and skills, including interventions, counselling, knowledge of drink/drugs interaction, research and evaluation. The practitioners should also have a solid theoretical background on the theories of substance misuse and addictive behaviour. The Department of Health report *Working in Partnership* (Department of Health 1994b) emphasises that mental health nurses encounter substance use problems as part of their workload and recommends that all mental health nurses should be capable of prevention, recognition and early intervention. The report also states that there is an urgent need to prepare mental health nurses and others in the primary health care teams to deal with substance misusers. In the National Alcohol Training Strategy report (Alcohol Concern 1994), it is stated

'. . . the basic training which is provided for professional staff such as doctors, nurses, social workers and probation officers ensures that they are competent in the performance of their professional role. It does not, however, always include the competencies required for the early identification of alcohol misuse, for offering appropriate response, and for making appropriate referrals where indicated. Professional staff also need opportunities for postbasic training to enable them to specialise in work with alcohol misusers.'

The All-Party Parliamentary Drug Misuse Group report (2000) recommended that:

'better training in substance misuse and dual diagnosis for doctors, nurses, social workers, probation officers, police and prison officers and voluntary sector personnel would assist in the early recognition of the condition and better accessibility to appropriate treatment provision.

The recent report of the working party of the Royal College of Psychiatrists (2000) suggested that both addiction and psychiatric services serve dual diagnosis poorly and consider that:

'the management of problem drug and alcohol misuse must become more central to the training of all mental health professionals, particularly those working in community psychiatric services.' (p. 233)

Crome (1999) argued that the substance misuse component should be integrated far more extensively into the undergraduate and postgraduate training programmes of mental health professionals.

Current status of educational programme

Despite these recommendations at national and international levels (WHO 1993), substance misuse components in the undergraduate medical, nursing, social work, pharmacy and psychology curricula lag behind current awareness of substance misuse as a major national health problem. Education about drugs and alcohol and their impact on health still find insufficient space within the medical curriculum (Glass 1988, 1990; Falkowski & Ghodse 1989) and that of pharmacy (Falkowski *et al.* 1989). In England, a review of the preparation of nurses at both preregistration and postregistration levels in substance misuse by the English National Board reaffirms the lack of adequate preparation of nurses, midwives and health visitors, the low priority accorded to substance misuse and the incongruity of curricular content (ENB 1995). The ENB recommends that substance use and misuse should be included in all preregistration and postregistration nursing, midwifery and health visiting curricular guidelines.

Falkowski and Ghodse (1990) reported that, on average, the amount of time devoted to alcohol-related disorders and drug dependence in adult nursing in the United Kingdom (UK) was 4.3 h, compared to 14.1 h for mental health nursing. This state of affairs is not solely restricted to the UK but also applies in Australia and the United States. A review of drug and alcohol content of nursing courses in Australia produced similar findings (Pols *et al.* 1993). Only 7% of the courses included 6 h or more of drug and alcohol-related education while an alarming 34% had no content related to drug and alcohol issues. Reviews of nursing curricula in the United States provide similar results, indicating the under-representation of substance misuse content in the nursing curricula (Murphy 1989; Hagemaster *et al.* 1993; Murphy-Parker & Rassool 2000). Sullivan and Handley (1992) identified that less than 5 h of substance misuse content is given in both Baccalaureate and Master's level nursing programmes. The paucity of substance misuse content in the curricula of undergraduate nursing courses is also common in Brazil (Villar-Luis *et al.* 2001) and other South American countries. Despite the recommendations, positional statements and educational initiatives in the US and UK (NNSA 1981; ENB 1995, 1996), there is little evidence to suggest that the integration of the substance misuse component in the undergraduate and postgraduate curriculum has been implemented in educational institutions (Happell & Taylor 1999; Rassool 1999, 2000). However, it is acknowledged that in the UK, the US and Australia the integration of substance use and misuse components in the undergraduate and postgraduate nursing curriculum are still restricted to a few centres of excellence.

The preparation of undergraduate medical students in substance use education is also limited in the medical curriculum. Paton's (1986) study, which examined formal teaching on alcohol in 26 medical schools, reveals that although all the schools provided some formal teaching about alcohol misuse, only one provided three formal sessions. Glass and Strang (1989) found that undergraduate medical students received, on average, 14 h of formal sessions in substance use with a mean of 6.7 h. In a recent survey of substance misuse education in British medical schools, Crome (1999) found that medical students are receiving 6 h of formal training and stated that the amount of input has halved since the early 1990s. However, she found that only one department within a medical school delivers 30 h of substance misuse education and coordinates another 30 h throughout the undergraduate medical education. Day *et al.* (1999) found that less than half of the respondents of 143 psychiatrists surveyed in the UK had received formal training in the management of substance misuse in the previous five years.

As regards social work and probation qualifying training, Harrison (1992, 1993a) suggested that there has been some improvement in integrating alcohol-related knowledge and skills in the curriculum. It seems that several social work courses are providing students with an extensive educational programme on substance use problems and in one case amounting to eight weeks of full-time formal education (Harrison 1993b).

Overall the progress in the integration of substance misuse the curriculum at undergraduate and postgraduate education in health and social care sciences has been limited.

New problem — new danger

Despite the magnitude of the problem, and even when substance use problems are identified, health care professionals may be reluctant to respond appropriately due to the lack of adequate preparation and negative attitudes towards substance misusers. Social prejudice, negative attitudes and stereotyped perceptions of substance misusers (Hanna 1991; Carroll 1996; Rassool 1998; Selleck & Redding 1998) and dual diagnosis patients (Williams 1999) are held widely amongst health care professionals and this may lead to minimal care being given to this population. Studies support that the development of a more positive and non-judgemental attitude and confidence and skills in identifying and working with substance misuse and related problems, may be partly related to the provision of education and training (Cartwright 1980; Hagemaster *et al.* 1993; Rassool 1993). However, much professional education and training reinforces the view that dealing with substance misuse is the job of a specialist (Rassool 1993, 2000). In the case of dual diagnosis patients, the responsibility for health and social care provisions is being shifted from one discipline to another and this 'diffusion of responsibility' is all too apparent.

Targeted training

Education and training in dual diagnosis, at a local level, should not be ad hoc but based upon a systematic planning. Initially, purchasers should develop an educational strategy with local authorities, educationalists and providers of services to identify the target needs and the planning of an educational programme. It is acknowledged that although this process is complex and time-consuming, it is invaluable in the delivering of high quality training and is service-driven. A training needs analysis is of paramount importance and should be part of a coherent strategy. The targeted audience should be mental health and addiction nurses, psychiatrists, social workers, prison health care staff, probation officers and others in the criminal justice system, primary health care teams and staff in the non-statutory organisations. In effect, all those who come into contact with dual diagnosis patients, generic and specialist staff, in both hospital and community settings should receive appropriate and regularly updated training. This question here is not who needs training in dual diagnosis but what kind and levels of training are required.

Level and content of educational programme

A systematic training need analysis with focus group interviews with selected disciplines and a content analysis of job specifications would provide an indication of the level of knowledge and competency required for a particular discipline. A two-tier model is proposed as shown in Table 17.1. The model includes both unidisciplinary and multidisciplinary educational programmes at basic and advanced levels. However, the core content to be included in an educational programme would undoubtedly depend on a number of factors such as the length of the course, its potential audience, the extent of prior learning and learning needs, and the nature of the course, either multi-professional or multi-disciplinary. It is argued that for generic personnel, a basic programme on substance misuse and mental health issues should be appropriate but with the consolidation of specific knowledge and

Table 17.1 Model of dual diagnosis educational programme

Type	Audience	Level	Content
Unidisciplinary	Generic	Basic	Attitudes and beliefs. Pattern of substance use and misuse. Types and effects of psychoactive substances. Screening & assessment (generic). Intervention strategies. Brief interventions. Physical health problems. Pregnancy, child protection and maternal health. HIV & Aids. Risk-reduction and prevention. Interaction of substance misuse and mental health. Suicide, violence & risk assessment. Care programme approach. Problems and issues in dealing with dual diagnosis patients. Models of care & management. Service models and provision. Self-help groups.
Multidisciplinary	Specialist	Advanced	Attitudes & beliefs. Diagnostic issues — DSM-IV & ICD. Substance misuse & psychiatric disorders — psychopathology. Epidemiology. Interactions effects of dual diagnosis. Ethical issues. Legislative framework. Prevention and risk reduction HIV & Aids. Personality disorders & violence. Crime. Suicide. Risk assessment. Child protection. Pregnancy and maternal health. Full assessment. Models of case management & treatment (substance misuse and mental health). Medication compliance. Shared care & care programme approach. Models of service provision. Relapse prevention. Motivational interviewing. Focus solution brief therapy. Health care needs assessment. Conceptual problems in research.

skills relevant to the particular discipline. For the specialist mental health workers, a more advanced programme should be instituted covering areas of advanced knowledge and therapeutic skills. The aims of the programme are to provide a more comprehensive knowledge and understanding of problems and issues related to substance use and mental health problems and to develop evidence-based interventions in clinical practice.

The principles of good practice in education and training and the design and delivery of training require the setting of clear aims, learning outcomes, content, teaching methodologies and evaluation. The teaching and learning strategies used should be innovative and these should be directed and guided by the learning outcomes. Visits and structured clinical placements should be incorporated as part of the educational plan. An important component in the design of the curriculum is the selection of tools and procedures to be used in the assessment of learning and the evaluation of the course. The challenge for educators and trainers in professional education is to change the educational paradigm from a traditional method of course development by adopting a framework based on the learning/occupational needs and innovative curriculum model.

Conclusion

In this chapter the emphasis has been on the importance of professional education and development on aspects of dual diagnosis. Professional development will always be most effective when it is part of a strategic plan to create an organisational learning culture (Rassool 1997).

There are challenges and barriers to overcome if we are to provide quality care to substance misusers and individuals with severe mental health problems or both.

The denial of health care workers and the general public alike of the existence of substance misuse continues to present an obstacle to the provision of early recognition, health education and effective care. Furthermore, health and social care professionals have a dissonance between their personal belief —therapeutic pessimism, that is there is nothing that can be done or should be done—and their professional roles (deskilled, lacking in confidence, etc.) (Rassool 2000). Another challenge is to overcome the marginalisation of the importance of substance misuse component in health and social care sciences curricula and clinical practice, at undergraduate and postgraduate levels. The consequences of lack of adequate education and training at all levels are a self-perpetuating cycle. Where a low priority is accorded to both policy and educational development in this area, there is no opportunity for health and social care professionals to develop role adequacy. This results in reinforcing the negative attitudes and the reluctance of health care professionals to respond effectively to substance misusers (Rassool 1993, 2000). Due to the nature and extent of dual diagnosis, a cultural shift is required in many of the paradigms that have traditionally guided the work of generic and specialist health and social care professionals.

References

Advisory Council on the Misuse of Drugs (1982) *Treatment and Rehabilitation*. HMSO, London

Advisory Council on the Misuse of Drugs (1988) *Aids and Drug Misuse. Part 1*. HMSO, London.

Advisory Council for the Misuse of Drugs (1989) *Aids and Drug Misuse. Part 2*. HMSO, London.

Advisory Council on the Misuse of Drugs (1990) *Problem Drug Use: A Review of Training*. HMSO, London.

Advisory Council on the Misuse of Drugs (1991) *Drug Misusers and the Criminal Justice System*. HMSO, London.

Alcohol Concern (1994) *A National Alcohol Training Strategy*. Alcohol Concern, London.

All-Party Parliamentary Drugs Misuse Group (2000) Report on Drug Misuse and Mental Health: Learning Lessons on Dual Diagnosis. April.

Carroll, J. (1996) Attitudes to drug users according to staff grade. *Professional Nurse* **11**, 718–720.

Cartwright, A. (1980) The attitude of helping agents towards the alcoholic client: the influence of experience, support, training and self-esteem. *British Journal of Addiction* **75**, 413–431.

Crome, I.B. (1999) The trouble with training: substance misuse training in British medical schools revisited. What are the issues? *Drugs: Education, Prevention and Policy* **6** (1), 111–123.

Day, E., Arcelus, J. & Kahn, A. (1999) Perceived role of psychiatrists in the management of substance misuse. A questionnaire survey. *Psychiatric Bulletin* **23** (11), 667–670.

Department of Health (1992) *Health of the Nation. A Strategy for Health in England*. HMSO, London.

Department of Health (1993) *The Health of the Nation. Key Area Handbook — Mental Illness*. HMSO, London.

Department of Health (1994a) *Tackling Drugs Together*. HMSO/Government Central Drugs Co-ordinating Unit, London.

Department of Health (1994b) *Working in Partnership: A Collaborative Approach to Care. A Report of the Mental Health Review Team*. HMSO, London.

English National Board for Nursing, Midwifery and Health Visiting (1995) Press Release. July. ENB, London.

English National Board for Nursing, Midwifery and Health Visiting (1996) *Substance Use and Misuse. Guidelines for Good Practice in Education and Training of Nurses, Midwives and Health Visitors*. ENB, London.

Falkowski, J. & Ghodse, A.H. (1989) Undergraduate medical school training in psychoactive drugs and rational prescribing in the United Kingdom. *British Journal of Addiction* **84**, 1339–1342.

Falkowski, J. & Ghodse, A.H. (1990) An international survey of the educational activities of schools of nursing on psychoactive drugs. *Bulletin of the World Health Organization* **68** (4), 479–482.

Falkowski, J., Ghodse, A.H., Dickinson, R. & Khan, I. (1989) An international survey of the educational activities of schools of pharmacy on psychoactive drugs. *Bulletin of the World Health Organization* **67** (5), 561–564.

Gafoor, M. & Rassool, G. Hussein (1998) The co-existence of psychiatric disorders and substance misuse: working with dual-diagnosis patients. *Journal of Advanced Nursing* **23** (3), 497–502.

Glass, I.B. (1988) Undergraduate training in substance abuse in the United Kingdom. *British Journal of Addiction* **84** (2), 197–202.

Glass, I.B. (1990) Alcohol misuse as a challenge to medical education: a belated remedy. *British Medical Bulletin* **50** (1), 164–170.

Glass, I.B. & Strang, J. (1989) Multiprofessional education in substance abuse in the UK and implications for training. World Health Organization Working Paper. WHO, London

Hagemaster, J., Handley, S., Plumlee, A., Sullivan, E. & Stanley, S. (1993) Developing educational programmes for nurses that meet today's addiction challenges. *Nurse Education Today* **13**, 421–425.

Hanna, Z.E. (1991) Attitudes towards problem drinkers revisited: patient–therapist factors contributing to the differential treatment of patients with alcohol problems. *Alcoholism: Clinical and Experimental Research* **15** (6), 927–931.

Happell, B. & Taylor, C. (1999) Drug and alcohol education for nurses: have we examined the whole problem. *Journal of Addictions Nursing* **11** (4), 180–185.

Harrison, L. (1992) Substance misuse and social work qualifying training in the British Isles: a survey of CQSW courses. *British Journal of Addiction* **87** (4), 635–642.

Harrison, L. (1993a) *Alcohol Problems: A Resource Directory and Bibliography*. Central Council for Education and Training in Social Work, London.

Harrison, L. (1993b) *Substance Misuse: Designing Social Work Training*. Central Council for Education and Training in Social Work, London.

Murphy, S.A. (1989) The urgency of substance abuse education in schools of nursing. *Journal of Nursing Education* **28**, 247–251.

Murphy-Parker, D. & Rassool, G. Hussein (2000) Education of Addictions in Nursing School Curriculum in the United States and the United Kingdom: The Urgent Need to Stir the Waters, Turn the Tide, Steer the Course and Effect a Change. Paper presented at the 25th National Nurses' Society on Addictions Education Conference, March 29 – April 2, 2000. Chicago.

National Nurses Society on Addictions (1981) Educating nurses on addiction. NNSA Position Paper. Raleigh, NC.

Paton, A. (1986) New survey of medical education. *Alcohol Concern* **2**, 14–16.

Pols, R.G., Cape, M.P., Ashenden, R. & Bush, R.A. (1993) *Proceedings: National Workshop Evaluation of Tertiary Education and Training on Alcohol and Drug Education*. National Centre for Education and Training on Addiction, Adelaide.

Rassool, G. Hussein (1993) Substance misuse: responding to the challenge. *Journal of Advanced Nursing* **18**, 9.

Rassool, G. Hussein (1997) Professional education and training. In: G.H. Rassool & M. Gafoor (eds) *Addiction Nursing: Perspectives on Professional and Clinical Practice*. Stanley Thornes (Publishers), Cheltenham.

Rassool, G. Hussein (1998) Contemporary issues in addiction nursing. In: G.H. Rassool (ed.) *Substance Use and Misuse: Nature, Context and Clinical Interventions*. Blackwell Science, Oxford.

Rassool, G. Hussein (1999) Substance use and misuse in nursing: beyond complacency. Editorial. *Association of Nurses in Substance Misuse (ANSA) Bulletin* **19** (1), 2.

Rassool, G. Hussein (2000) Addiction: global problem and global response complacency or commitment? Guest Editorial *Journal of Advanced Nursing* **32** (3), 505–508.

Royal College of Psychiatrists, & Royal College of Physicians (2000) *Drugs: Dilemmas and Choices*. Gaskell, London.

Selleck, C.S. & Redding, B.A. (1998) Knowledge and attitudes of registered nurses towards perinatal substance abuse. *Journal of Obstetric, Gynaecologic and Neonatal Nursing* **27**, 70–78.

Sullivan, E.J. & Handley, S.M. (1992) Alcohol and drug abuse in nurses. *Annual Review of Nursing Research* **10**, 113–125.

Villar-Luis, M., Pillon, S. & Rassool, G. Hussein (2001) Substance use in the nursing curriculum: the Brazilian experience. Unpublished Paper.

Williams, K. (1999) Attitudes of mental health professionals to co-morbidity between mental health problems and substance misuse. *Journal of Mental Health* **8** (6), 606–613.

World Health Organization (1993) WHO Expert Committee on Drug Dependence. *28th Report*. WHO, Geneva.

Index